50 Athletes Over 50 Teach Us to Live a Strong, Healthy Life

Tools, Insights, and Inspiration for Living Spectacularly

by Don McGrath Ph.D.

The author is grateful for the expert submissions of Nikola Medic, Ph.D., and Vonda Wright, M.D.

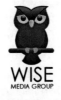

WISE
MEDIA GROUP

Wise Media Group
Denver, CO

This book is dedicated to those who aspire to live a strong, healthy life that is full of fun and adventure.

Foreword

I know of no other book that speaks so well to those who want to continue to ply their exercise as they age. Based on interviews with 50 athletes over 50, this work offers valuable insights into how older individuals successfully maintain regular exercise and sports programs.

Spellbinding, inspirational stories of consistency and accomplishment are the lynchpins of this book. Their bold lives provide joy and satisfaction, and greater health and stamina is their prize.

Banana George Blair, age 94
World-famous barefoot water skier

The Crowd Cheers

I am ever grateful to the athletes that I interviewed for this book, who so graciously volunteered their time and personal energy to this project. Their counsel and encouragement were absolutely invaluable.

My wife Sylvia deserves a ton of thanks for supporting me. During the time I worked on this book, Sylvia was starting her own business. We have both been very busy, but never so busy that we missed a step in our wonderful relationship.

Due, in part, to my coaches, teammates and climbing partners, I have had a life full of exhilarating movement. Many thanks to each of them. They deserve appreciation for inspiring me, pushing me, and creating an environment that helped me succeed in my chosen sports.

I am very thankful that I came to know Brian Schwartz, who led me through the 50 Interviews process and who was the catalyst for this book. His program opened up possibilities for me that I could never have imagined.

I appreciate Rue Smith and Tracy Monthei, who helped me jumpstart the 50-K Active/Athletic Challenge. The Challenge, which serves to recruit 50,000 people to adopt five healthy athletic habits, was inspired by the athletes featured in this book.

How grateful I am to Nikola Medic, Ph.D., for his internationally known research contributions in sports psychology. His vantage point of many years of observation and counseling with masters athletes and with athletic teams provides a unique perspective.

I feel fortunate to have enlisted support from Vonda Wright, M.D., whose well known expertise on the performance of aging athletes added a great deal to my knowledge. Her words both inspire and inform.

My great appreciation to my editor Karen Hart, who helped me hone my message.

Special thanks go to Sharon Pearson, whose keen proofreading eye helped polish the rough.

Finally, I wish to thank my sisters Mary Ann, Kathy, Gerri and Donna, who carry on the spirit of our parents by staying near and supporting me.

Table of Contents

The Warm Up

My wake-up call came in the form of a medical check-up that I had in my mid-thirties when I complained to my doctor about lower back pain, acid reflux, and a few other small ailments. As he responded to me half-jokingly that I was "on schedule," I started to realize that maybe I needed to take better care of myself. It turned out, that with a little physical therapy and a tweak to my diet, I felt better. In fact, by the time I hit 40, I felt better than I had since my late twenties.

The value of that medical exam was that, clearly, whatever exercise and health care measures had worked in my twenties would not carry me through my forties and beyond. I needed to employ new strategies if I was going to continue to maintain excellent health.

When I met Brian Schwartz, who created the company 50 Interviews, Inc., I found a way to uncover these strategies. Brian's concept is that authors select a topic that they are passionate about and interview 50 people who are successful in that area. By surrounding myself with individuals over age 50 that I admired, I could build a network of people who were adept at sustaining strength and wellness throughout the years. This would ensure my own success. The ideas found in this book represent information and lessons gathered from my interviews with 50 athletes over 50 years old. Their experiences and insights are useful for people of all ages.

I knew there must be some way to keep enjoying good health through physical activity in the important later years of my life. What mindset or approaches did I need to use? Even a casual look at athletes in their forties, fifties, sixties and beyond, made me believe that we can continue to make progress with our exercise, and in some cases yield big returns from sports, well after what would be considered over the hill. Could it be that we expect too little of ourselves?

Initially, my goal in writing this book was to understand the challenges facing older athletes who tend to train less, which results in a drop in their performance. I hoped to uncover some insights into how some of them keep at it and perform at high levels. However, I soon realized that this book would become much more than that. My subjects taught me lessons that shifted my focus from athletic performance, to something else that allows us to live a strong and healthy life as we age.

Having developed a list of interview questions, I began my search for 50 athletes over 50. I first posted to a forum on Geezerjock.com, asking for volunteers who were willing to be interviewed. Ken Stone of Mastertrack.com noticed the post, and when he wrote about it in his blog, I received many inquiries. At the same time, I found a few athlete profiles on Geezerjock. com that looked hopeful, so I sent messages to Sandy Scott, Carl Bamforth, Terry Peterson, and Linda Quirk. Before I knew it, I had a dance card full of interviews and my job was to keep up with my new schedule.

Unfortunately, due to limited space, I was not able to include detailed interviews of all the over-50 athletes. Their stories are also very valuable to the discussion about sustaining a healthy life, and you can find their full interviews at www.50athletesover50.com.

One of the things that I learned was that when we pass our twenties, those of us who were involved in sports face a major challenge. It becomes harder to access organized teams, workout facilities, and coaches, which is what we depend on for optimal training. And the importance of optimal training is, of course, what allows us to be highly competitive. We are then at a loss, since when we were young, being competitive was our orientation.

After doing only 15 interviews, I realized that these older athletes share a common set of characteristics that carry them through their later years. The critical piece that came to light over and over again was that to continue to reap the benefits of an active life as we age, we must transition from having a performance focus to a lifestyle focus. What does this mean? Unlike younger athletes, older athletes are not usually as interested in performance and competition, but have a much broader perspective.

Their most important goal typically changes from performance, to wanting to be active for a long time. There are other common characteristics as well. Most say that they want to have good health, enjoy their sport, and have fun with their athletic friends! They also work at being injury free, since as we get older, recovery from injuries is slower.

To support these new priorities, they envision exercise or a sport, to which they are committed. Some may have the ability to envision goals that seem out of the ordinary. If so, they firmly, carefully and consistently, integrate that activity into their lifestyle. With a high level of passion that comes from practicing their exercise, they see their physical activity as play, rather than work.

Additionally, many of the athletes that I spoke with are examples of the growing awareness that with the right focus, our bodies are capable of more than we think. Based on my interviews, it appears that athletes like Dara Torres, who competes at world class levels beyond the age of 40, are not just a curiosity. They are examples that aging can be influenced by the active lifestyle we choose.

As I discovered the fascinating stories of my subjects and the parallels between them, I couldn't wait for my alarm clock to go off each morning so that I could meet more athletes over-50. This was truly a life-changing experience, because I was immersing myself in a widening pool of knowledge developed by resilient, older athletes, who demonstrate their fitness every single day.

What I learned from the over-50 athletes is invaluable to me, as it will certainly help me to secure an active lifestyle in the future. I believe that the knowledge that they shared is a great asset to anyone who wants to sustain a healthy, active life.

Chapter 1:
A Strong Healthy Life

"Today is life – the only life you are sure of. Make
the most of today. Get interested in something.
Shake yourself awake. Develop a hobby. Let the
winds of enthusiasm sweep through you.
Live today with gusto."

-Dale Carnegie

A compilation of striking stories of 50 athletes over 50 years old, this book is designed to help us understand how exercise and sports can continue to help us lead strong, healthy lives as we age. In the larger context of exercising throughout life, the athletes that I interviewed prove that while staying fit as we age differs from when we were younger, it is critical and can yield astounding results.

In this work, I will refer interchangeably to athletes as people who exercise, or as people who participate in a sport. Although some may think of athletes as masters of a sport or game, a truer definition is a "person who is trained or skilled in exercises, sports or games requiring physical strength, agility or stamina." Many of the athletes I interviewed participate in sports, but not all. Some engage in non-competitive physical activities that

1

yield the same benefits. The key is to have an activity that you love; one that engages your muscles and gets your heart and lungs pumping.

So, what is a strong, healthy life? Good health underscores a strong life, and to be strong is to be powerful, vigorous, courageous, and stable. A strong life is one of confidence and capabilities; one in which challenges and adventures are taken on without undue fear and anxiety. A strong life is full of fun and adventure and when done fully, is spectacular.

Physical activity not only strengthens the body, but when coupled with goals, creates a powerful brew that strengthens the will and our overall ability to accomplish what we set out to do. I am excited to share with you many older athletes who are living strong, and yes, spectacular lives. You will meet Linda Quirk, who ran seven marathons on seven continents and plans to run across four of the world's biggest deserts. Linda does these feats not for herself, but to raise money for a good cause. You will read about Sandy Scott, an astounding cyclist with a remarkable "comeback" history. You will read about Myrna Haag, a talented triathlete with a mission to change people's lives in her community by helping them break their food addictions.

If you are exercising, maybe this book will challenge you to more vigorous activity. If you have quit exercising, I hope this book encourages you to begin again. If you aren't exercising, maybe you will be inspired to start. As we'll see, it truly is never too late for exercise to make a serious difference in our lives, and the benefits for older adults are more dramatic than you may have imagined.

Health Benefits of an Active Life

Health benefits of an active life are not just nice to have – they often make the difference between just getting by and living a life of high quality and independence. The leading cause of death in America is cardiovascular disease, and studies show that age is the major risk factor. And according to John Raty, MD, author of the book *Spark: The Revolutionary New Science of Exercise and the Brain*, cancer and stroke follow heart disease as leading causes of death in those over 65. He adds that this trio represents 61 percent of deaths in that age group.

Nonetheless, we have at our fingertips, an enormously powerful weapon against these and many other diseases. The following facts and statements barely scratch the surface of this topic, but show the heartening impact that regular exercise has on many different diseases.

According to the American Heart Association, physical inactivity is the primary cause of heart disease.

A classic study on the improvement in longevity through regular lifetime physical activity, showed that physical fitness and exercise can reduce the risk of diseases such as heart disease, non-insulin-dependent diabetes mellitus, some cancers, osteoarthritis, osteoporosis and obesity.[1]

An American Cancer Society study on breast cancer found that although any physical activity appeared to have some benefit, a 30 percent reduction in breast cancer rate occurred in women whose exercise was the equivalent of swimming, running, or jogging at least six hours a week.[2]

The University of Utah and Kaiser Permanente in Oakland, California, found that men and women lowered their risk of colorectal cancer with exercise, and that vigorous exercise provided the greatest benefit. Men and women who exercised the equivalent of jogging five or more hours a week, lowered their risk 40 to 50 percent.

A follow-up to a Harvard study found that the women of a group with diabetes who exercised at least four hours a week, were 40 percent less likely to develop heart disease.[3] Other studies have found similar trends for men.

In support of these statements, it became obvious early on in my interview process that exercise and training routines of those I interviewed were having an enormous effect on their health. While more than 60 percent of U.S. adults over the age of 20 are overweight or obese, there are only one or two athletes in my group that are overweight – and none are obese.

According to the Center for Disease Control (CDC), the average American goes to the doctor's office three times per year, and 18 percent of their visits are for prevention. The over-50 athletes reported about the same number of offices visits, but nearly 60 percent of them were preventative in nature. The CDC notes that the most common conditions seen in office visits are hypertension (high blood pressure) at 28 percent, arthritis at 17.5 percent and diabetes at 12 percent. The occurrence of these conditions in my group of athletes was much lower; hypertension four percent, arthritis four percent and diabetes two percent.

Other research shows that emotional well-being and a higher quality of life are other important byproducts of physical activity. It is common knowledge that exercise releases endorphins in the brain, which makes us feel good. In addition, there's great value in being strong and healthy as a means of living independently and more constructively as we age. Consider these statements:

Dr. Lakatta, MD, senior investigative chief, Laboratory of Cardiovascular Science at the National Institute on Aging says, "Emerging scientific evidence suggests that people who exercise regularly not only live longer, they live better. Studies also show that exercise can promote psychological well-being and reduce feelings of anxiety and depression."

In his book Spark: The Revolutionary New Science of Exercise and the Brain, *Dr. Raty tells us that exercise is the best defense against mood disorders and Alzheimer's disease.*

Director of the National Institute on Aging, Richard J. Hodes, MD says, "Cardiovascular disease is also a major cause of disability, limiting the activity and eroding the quality of life of millions of older people each year."

Still, there is even good news for those who aren't currently active. Exercise can boost cardiac fitness in out-of-shape older people as well as conditioned older people. According to Dr. Lakatta, who was the principal investigator of a 1996 study on aerobic exercise for sedentary, older people, "... aerobic exercise conditioning can offset normal aging of the heart by making it a better pump, even for those who begin later in life, at age 60 or 70...*a novel aspect of this study found that the relative benefits were the same regardless of how fit they were when they started exercising.*"

That's encouraging for any of us who are out-of-shape, but there is another challenge to address; how do we handle the significant, undisputed effects of chronological aging on our bodies? The changes that occur in all of our body's systems affect our ability to participate in sports and other vigorous physical activities. Effects seen in typical healthy adults can be quite dramatic, and include loss of muscle mass and tone, loss of aerobic endurance, loss of muscular power, increase in body fat, and an overall decrease in functional capacity to do physical work.

We need to keep in mind as we review these changes, that although they can sound daunting, they can be managed. *With the exception of decreased maximum heart rate, studies have found that almost all physiological changes in older people can be counteracted by athletic training.*

Scientific reports show that after our late twenties or early thirties, we lose about 10 percent of our aerobic capacity each decade, up to age 60 or 70, at which time it decreases at a much faster rate.[4] Studies of masters endurance athletes indicate that peak performance can be maintained until 35 years of age, with a modest reduction in performance thereafter, up to age 60 or 70. The main reason for the decline is a decrease in maximal aerobic capacity (Vo2 max), somewhat related to a reduced maximum heart rate.

Additionally, the muscle mass that we lose as we age causes a reduction in our ability to generate power. We also lose muscle fibers, called fast twitch fibers, which enable powerful movement. On a side note, loss of muscle mass contributes significantly to the slowdown of metabolism, and also to the commensurate increase in body fat that we have as we get older. Now along with age-related changes, comes another potential pitfall.

Staying Injury Free

Athlete or not, as we age we all feel the effects of slower recovery, either from injury or from overdoing it. One of the major effects of aging is that our body becomes less effective at repairing itself. I like to draw an analogy between our life cycle and that of a building. During the first couple decades, our building is being constructed. The frame, the exterior, and wiring are all being installed and refined. A huge amount of energy is expended, and many workers are involved in this phase.

Once the building is complete, the effects of wear and tear begin to show. The maintenance crew takes over, and begins to make repairs to the many things that begin to break down. As the building ages, not only does the building develop problems, but the repairmen also age. They don't do quite as good of a job as they did when they were younger.

Unfortunately, it's not as simple as firing the repairmen and replacing them with ones that are more able. Physical training does help the repairmen stay sharp, but it has two opposing effects. On one hand, training improves our body's ability to repair itself by improving circulation and other body functions. It is well known that a person who is fit will most likely recover from surgery faster than someone who is unfit. On the other hand, training puts more wear and tear on our bodies, and exposes us to injury.

The Main Reason for Age-Related Decrease in Exercise

While staying injury free is obviously important to sustained athletics, what is the main reason for a decrease in exercise capability as we age? Looking at the broad range of studies, it appears that it is due to socio-behavioral changes.[5] With age, we tend to train less frequently, consistently or intensely.

Typical reasons for training less are job and family responsibilities. Such socio-behavioral reasons for training less are prevalent, but they are not a given. We can see this with the 50 athletes I interviewed who have managed to stay very active. Most cherish balance as an important component to a successful life. The result is that they keep their exercise schedules, as well as their work and family relationships, intact. In the chapters that follow we will see how the athletes accomplish this.

Despite the effects of chronological aging, greater susceptibility to injury and temptation to put other aspects of life ahead of sports and exercise, the evidence is overwhelming that running our engines hot protects us from the onset of many illnesses and promotes a sense of well-being. Those of us who have found this empirically may not know the statistics, but we understand at some level, that being active is very important for our welfare.

It is possible to live a healthy life without being strong, but not the converse. Exercise is a powerful pill!

[1]Paffenbarger, R. 1996. "Physical Activity and Fitness for Health and Longevity." *Research Quarterly for Exercise and Sports*, Vol. 67, No.3: 11-3.

[2]Patel, Alpa, PhD. *Cancer Causes and Control*. Vol. 14, No. 6: 519-529.

[3]Hu, Frank B., MD; Stampfer, Meir J., MD; Solomon, Caron, MD; Liu, Simin, MD; Colditz, Graham A., MD; Speizer, Frank E., MD; Willett, Walter C., MD; and Manson, JoAnn E., MD. January 16, 2001. "Physical Activity and Risk for Cardiovascular Events in Diabetic Women." *Annals of Internal Medicine*. Vol. 134, No. 2: 96-105. Harvard School of Public Health.

[4]Taylor, Albert W.; Johnson, Michael, J., MD. 2008. "Physiology of Exercise and Healthy Aging". *Human Kinetics*.

[5]Tanaka, H., Seals, D.R. 2003. "Dynamic Exercise Performance in Masters Athletes: Insight into Effects of Primary Human Aging on Physiological Functional Capacity." *Journal of Applied Physiology* 95: 2152-2162.

Chapter 2:
The Performance-to-Lifestyle Transition

*"I still get wildly enthusiastic about little things...
I play with leaves. I skip down the street and run
against the wind."*

-Leo Buscaglia

When I began the interview process, I had a very different view of what it means to be an older athlete than I do today. The year before I started work on this book, I developed a workshop aimed at helping busy professionals achieve their sports goals. I crafted the diagram in *Figure 1* (as can be seen on following page) to illustrate the components of sports performance.

The figure shows that to achieve high performance, an athlete needs to find the right mix of physical and mental fitness, technique, nutrition, goals, and the ability to execute at the right time. Individuals may choose to focus on the aspects that suit them best and yield optimum results. This simplistic, mechanistic model was taught by coaches and trainers in my teens and through college. At the time, I thought that it made sense for athletes of all ages.

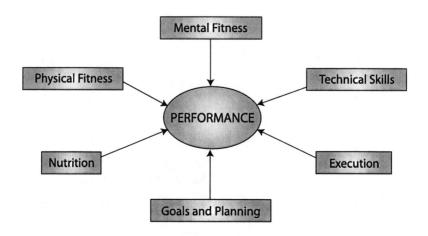

Figure 1: The Original Performance Focused Model

After I completed most of the interviews with the 50 over-50 athletes, I realized that this model didn't reflect the world in which this older group lives. This model may very well work for younger athletes, whose focus tends to be on learning their sport and being as competitive as they can be. Yet it doesn't apply very well to many of the older athletes I interviewed.

I would bet that if you asked high school or college-age athletes about their ultimate achievements, they would nearly all recount winning a race, setting a record, or something related to performance. Yet 40 percent of the over-50 athletes who I spoke with said that their biggest accomplishment would be to continue their exercise or sport for a long time. They are not as concerned with performance; their main goal is to keep at it for as long as they can, so they can live a strong, healthy life.

I call this passage where older athletes, and sometimes younger athletes, often go from being performance-focused to having a broader perspective on exercise and health, the Performance-to-Lifestyle Transition. Even though the transition is more common in older athletes, athletes of any age can work through it. During the process, older athletes substitute different motivators for performance, while younger athletes who are making this passage, may adopt some of those motivators as well.

Regarding high performance, some older athletes continue to be motivated by competitive performance. They are the ones who can envision out of the ordinary goals and persevere to win awards. Their accomplishments are stunning, especially given their ages. Yet, these athletes also have a keener appreciation than most of their younger counterparts, for fitness benefits that go beyond athletic achievements.

Performance-to-Lifestyle Transition Phases

To help us understand how the transition works, I developed the model in *Figure 2*, again based on my interviews of the 50 athletes over 50. In this transition model there are three key phases: *Dream It, Live It,* and *Love It*; and the first, *Dream It*, is central.

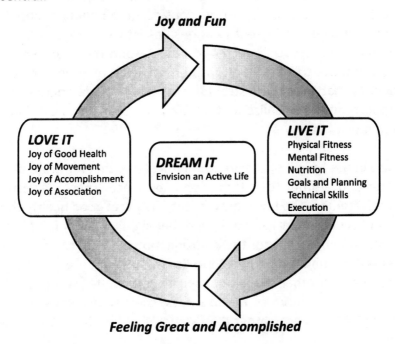

Figure 2: The Performance-to-Lifestyle Model

Dream It

In the *Dream It* phase, athletes envision themselves as being fulfilled, healthy and happy, due to an active lifestyle. They see themselves exercising consistently and being committed to regular physical activity. Some stretch their imaginations and visualize accomplishing goals that are outside of the norm. This kind of possibility thinking is important, because without it, there can be no accomplishment. As children, we knew how to stretch our imaginations. How many of us wanted to be cowboys, or princesses, or astronauts, or race car drivers? Even better, was when our neighbor's son thought outside of the usual box when he said that he wanted to be an insurance salesman when he grew up. And my wife once told me that she had wanted to be a cow when she was a kid. Now that's possibility thinking!

Love It

The *Love It* phase encompasses the opportunity to play, to have fun. In our society it may be hard to find fun, as we strive to achieve at work, earn what we consider to be enough money, and find time to keep our relationships intact. Maybe we have a little time to socialize, maybe not. Despite these pressures, Performance-to-Lifestyle Transition athletes revel in physical activity that gives them strength and health, while offering the opportunity to socialize and have a good time. Who can have too much fun?

Also in the *Love It* phase are four critical joys that motivate athletes and prompt their transition experience. These powerful motivators are the joy of movement, the joy of good health, the joy of achievement, and the joy of belonging to a group of like-minded people. It is for these strong motivators that older athletes don't find it very difficult to do hard workouts, eat right, or make time for their exercise or sports. Even better, when focusing on one or more of the four joys, exercise becomes something that they are, rather than something that they do.

As we will see, the *Love It* motivators wield great influence. They help compensate for the changes in our bodies and minds that take place as we age, of which can stop us from being active. Alleviating those changes allows us to more successfully navigate the Performance-to-Lifestyle Transition.

Live It

The *Live It* phase includes physical fitness, mental fitness, technical skills, execution, and goals. These traits represent the nuts and bolts of what we need to do to remain healthy and achieve whatever level of strength or expertise we want. The four joys are critical to the *Live It* step, because they provide the motivation to put fitness, exercise plans, etc. to use. When athletes employ these traits, feelings of satisfaction based on good health and accomplishment are generated, and these feelings cycle back to further feed joy in the *Love It* phase.

The feedback and interaction between having the joys of an active life, and the physical exercise that creates these joys, form a powerful flywheel that energizes people and helps them stay in the game. Successful completion of the Performance-to-Lifestyle Transition is defined by the point at which this flywheel reaches an energy level that sustains athletes through the many challenges to staying active.

The Four Joys as Motivators and How They Change

The four joys in the *Love It* phase help the over-50 athlete manage physical and mental changes, and also provide strong incentives for exercise and sports. It is helpful to know what they are, which are most important, and what to expect from them. It also helps to know that the intensity of the joys can change as we age.

In my survey, I found that 41 percent of the 50 athletes were most motivated by the joy of movement, or play. Next, 38 percent were most motivated by the joy of good health, nine percent by the joy of achievement, and 12 percent the joy of association. The joys hold the key to continued engagement in exercise for older adults, so understanding them is important for a strong, healthy life.

The Joy of Good Health

Younger athletes often drive themselves, and give little thought to the health benefits from physical activities. That is, unless they suffer an injury or minor illness from the stress put on their bodies. As we reach our forties, we notice that because we are active, our health is superior to our less-active contemporaries.

This observation is a strong motivator, because about that time we start seeing less-active friends and relatives become out-of-shape, or even develop chronic or life-threatening diseases. The athletes who make the Performance-to-Lifestyle Transition are more intent on keeping their strength and good health as they age. The joy of good health is a powerful motivating factor that keeps that flywheel going.

The Joy of Movement

When we are young, we delight in moving our bodies. Play is inherent in children and they have the instinct to move. They are also naturally motivated to learn new games and skills. For adults too, playfulness spurs the joy of movement. It is well-known that when we move, especially strenuously, for long periods of time, endorphins are activated in our brains and give us a sense of well-being.

As we age, the play instinct is challenged in several ways. We become overwhelmed with other priorities, and not knowing how to integrate playfulness into our lives, it falls by the wayside. In addition, those who have been involved with one activity for many years often become tired of it, and lose that playful spirit. If we do remain active, we begin to appreciate that while it's not as easy as it used to be, we still love the sensation of physical play and the pleasure that we get from it.

In Stuart Brown's book *Play*, he explains that one aspect of play is that it is engaging, and when we are deeply engaged in play we lose track of time. If through exercise we tap into our instinct to play, we find that our workout flies by. At that point, there is no other place in the world that we would rather be.

The Joy of Achievement

We all love to achieve something that we have worked hard for. In individual exercise, we are likely to be pleased with greater stamina, longer workouts, and greater expertise. In a sport, we may enjoy seeing a higher level of performance, be it faster times, better distances, etc.

However, as we age, performance gradually degrades and we experience some regression. This difficulty causes many people to abandon an active life. What makes a difference for most successful Performance-to-Lifestyle Transition athletes is that they are satisfied to de-emphasize high performance and identify with other motivators.

Apart from altering their definition of accomplishment, it helps athletes who are transitioning to a lifestyle focus, to change their exercise, or to create an adventure around their activity. For example, they can switch from swimming to running, or make their sport an adventure by entering in an athletic meet at a place they've been interested in visiting. Changing their outlook, and using these incentives, rejuvenates their joy of achievement, which motivates them to keep working out.

The Joy of Association

People who have belonged to a team or group that regularly workout together know what a great experience it can be. I cherish my memories of being on my high school and college cross-country teams, and I remain in contact with some of my former teammates to this day. When we leave school behind, launch a career, and possibly start a family, we can lose association with active contemporaries. When that happens, we often lose and miss the sense of belonging to a group of athletic, like-minded people.

Thriving Performance-to-Lifestyle athletes manage to maintain a connection with an active fitness-oriented community. For these people, the connection becomes a priority, because it offers them a support network that helps them continue to live an active life. Options for associating with other active people include seeking individuals to share exercise with, associating with others in gym classes, joining a walking or running group, or joining a sports team or club.

All of the over-50 athletes that I interviewed have successfully made the Performance-to-Lifestyle Transition using the four joys. In doing so, they are happily reaping the benefits of a strong, healthy life.

Approaches to Exercise

I find that the athletes I studied were in three categories, and the categories are defined by the approaches they used to stay active.

I call the first and largest group, the Innovators, which comprise 47 percent of those surveyed. They don't hesitate to change their sport – sometimes more than once – to keep their physically active life fresh and interesting. Bloomers, the second category, represent 32 percent of the athletes, and they take up a sport later in life with the goal of being healthier. Definitely in a groove, I call the last category Groovers. They focus primarily on one sport from their youth and throughout their adult life. Representing only 21 percent of those surveyed, they are in the minority.

The fact that the majority of the over-50 athletes are in the Innovators group leads me to believe that shifting from one sport to another and maybe another again, is a viable approach to staying fit longer. Altering sports is a refreshing opportunity to use different muscles, create interest, meet new people, and to frequent new locations. Such stimulating change promotes growth and keeps them engaged.

The Innovators you will meet include Dave Dyc and Maria Riquet. They changed from the sport that they were once dedicated to for a variety of reasons. Dave shifted from surfing to outrigger canoeing because he loved the beauty of his surroundings and because he liked the workout it gave him. Following a horrible bicycle accident, Maria took up weight lifting and bodybuilding.

Bloomers I interviewed include Cheryl Ragsdale and Merrill Schwartz. At age 48, Cheryl stumbled on boxing and martial arts and is now working toward a black belt. To control his weight, Merrill started running in his mid-thirties. He now participates in triathlons and endurance cycling adventures.

Athletes Jane Welzel and Ward Smith are examples of Groovers. Groovers remind me somewhat of Malcolm Gladwell's book *Outliers* and the people he calls by that name. Gladwell's outliers are people who are extremely successful in their chosen field, and they include Bill Gates and The Beatles.

So what do Groovers have in common with outliers? Gladwell suggests that outliers are people who were lucky because they happened upon their passion at an opportune time in history. In addition, they were able to spend over 10,000 hours immersed in their pursuit.

While Jane and Ward may not be as successful as Bill Gates or The Beatles, they have managed to pull off the relatively rare feat of participating in one sport for, what is up to now, their entire lives. The athletes I interviewed reported an average weekly workout time of seven hours. So, considering that the athletes I studied are over-50 years old and have likely devoted seven hours a week or more to working out, Groovers most certainly have surpassed Gladwell's 10,000-hour threshold. With this kind of single-minded focus, Groovers develop the desire and discipline to practice their sport or exercise regularly and intensely, even as they age.

Innovator, Bloomer and Groover Interviews

The interviews that follow are examples of innovators, bloomers and groovers, who have successfully made the Performance-to-Lifestyle Transition.

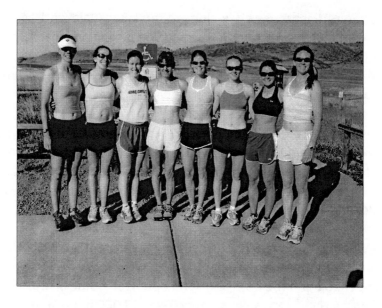

Jane Welzel (fourth from left) and her running friends.

"For me, success now means that I am fit enough, healthy enough, and capable of enjoying running."
- Jane Welzel

Groover Jane Welzel is a 54-year-old distance runner who lives in Fort Collins, Colorado. Originally from Hopkinton, Massachusetts, where the Boston marathon begins, Jane has kept her New England accent despite living elsewhere for many years.

She has participated in a long list of sports since her childhood including, field hockey, gymnastics, basketball, tennis, swimming, water polo, crew, cross-country, road racing, and track. Quite by chance, Jane took up running, and it was to become her long-term sport. She was involved in this sport before the women's running boom of the 1970s, but the boom did influence her running history.

At the start of her junior year at the University of Massachusetts, Jane was planning to continue to be on the swim team. Fortunately, when she arrived on campus, two things conspired to put her in touch with the sport that she will practice for the rest of her life. One was that the pool was under repair. The other was that the school had just added women's cross-country as a sport in response to Title IX legislation. This legislation required, in part, that any athletic program that received federal financial assistance must offer the same kinds of opportunities for women as for men.

Without a swimming pool, and not wanting to get out of shape, Jane started running with the cross-country team. Two weeks later at the first meet, she was the school's top runner. She went on to qualify for five Olympic trials in the marathon, run as a professional, and coach at the college level.

In addition to making running an integral part of her life, Jane also pays it forward to her running community. She is very involved in organizing races and holds workouts every week, drawing runners of all abilities. She plans to run for the rest of her life because she just loves to run.

Q: Tell me what it was like to be involved early in the women's running movement.

A: It was 1984, and those of us working on it had just got the marathon added as an Olympic event. We had proved through the Avon racing series that women all over the world could race the marathon, and that it deserved to be in the Olympics.

That year, the Olympic marathon trials were such a big deal for women runners. I can't explain how emotional it was just to be there. On the day I was in the trials, I ran my personal record of around 2:35. I finished 14th among the best women in the country.

Those first Olympic trials were my springboard. Through them I found out I was a good runner, so I decided that I would find out what it was like to be a professional. Unfortunately, within six months of the trial I broke my neck in a bad car accident. After that, the 1988 Olympic trials were special to me because participating in them became my goal after the accident.

I broke my neck in December 1984, and in late April on my birthday, I had my sister take me to the track so I could try to run a mile. I thought I could run 7:30, and my sister paced me perfectly at a 7:27. I remember looking at her and saying that I just needed to run 25 more of those back-to-back, about 90 seconds per mile faster.

I had three years until the trials, and I thought I could do it. And I did! I qualified for the 1988 trials, finishing 13th at an amazing 2:36. This was basically the same place and same time I had achieved during the 1984 trials before I broke my neck.

Q: How do you feel about competition now that you are older?

A: For some people, competition is the big thing, and when they can't be competitive, their desire to train goes away. I've always found a way to include running as part of my whole lifestyle. Competing doesn't drive me, but participation does. Plus, I enjoy helping to put on events and I enjoy participating in them. I put on two races every year, and that is a way for me to give back to something that has given me a lot of pleasure.

Q: What are the keys to your success?

A: I would answer this question differently if I was asked this many years ago. I define success differently now. The keys to my success now mean that I am fit enough, healthy enough, and capable of enjoying running. I have a group of women that I run with three times per week. Most are younger than me, so I like being able to run with them because they keep me in shape. I organize weekly workouts that bring people of all abilities together who share the passion for running.

Q: What was the best advice you were ever given?

A: It would be that I'm not defined by my running. I was thinking that if I ran well, that meant something, or if I didn't run well, that meant something. Pete Pfitzinger straightened me out when we were out on a run one day. I was complaining that I didn't feel prepared for some race, and he told me to go back and look at my log book, and see that I had done the work. He also said that all you can do is go and run the best race that you can, and that is good enough.

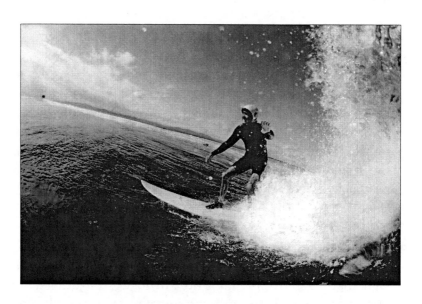

Ward Smith catching a wave!

"Surf now!"

- Ward Smith

Groover Ward Smith is a 61-year-old surfer from Aptos, California, which is in the Santa Cruz Mountains. Ward came from an active and resourceful family. He remembers water skiing when he was six years old, although his family didn't own a boat. Ward's father knew lots of people, and the family got to take part in many fun activities that influenced Ward's life. Living very near the beach gave Ward lots of opportunity to participate in water sports. He has many fond memories of surfing on rubber mats at Huntington Beach when he was seven years old.

Ward remembers going to see surfer movies like *Gidget* and the movies made by Bud and Bruce Brown, and he'd come home buzzing. Watching these movies and loving the water made Ward want to learn to surf, and his parents were very supportive. When he bought his first surf board, they all had fun with it, first in the pool and then at the beach. He remembers the first time that he went to the beach to surf with his new board. Not knowing that waves in the ocean weren't constant and had to be spotted, he ended up just hilariously sitting on his board in calm water; never catching a single wave.

Ward has surfed ever since. He has even molded his career around his love of surfing. He first taught in the California public schools for a number of years, but 18 years ago he began working with other teachers and parents to form Alternative Family Education, which administers homeschooling. Ward loves teaching at the alternative school, which gives him more flexibility to surf more often when surfing is good.

Q: It sounds like you surf a lot. How often do you surf?
A: As much as I can. I surfed over 160 days per year over the past two years. I don't mind surfing in less than ideal conditions. I've surfed when the water was 48 degrees and the air was 34 degrees. That's commitment!

Q: What are your surfing goals?

A: They aren't your typical goals. My goal is just to surf as much as I can. I want to surf the good waves and to continue to surf the best that I can. I can still surf the short boards, which are harder to paddle, take more energy to get into the waves, and are more difficult to use. I want to surf waves to around 12 feet high, which I still feel comfortable with. One day I was sitting on a cliff watching the swell, and the conditions weren't great. It hit me that regardless, I needed to get out there. I now have the license plate "SURF NOW."

Q: What things do you believe differentiate you from your contemporaries who have tailed off in their athletic participation and abilities?

A: I love hanging out with the other surfers, no matter how old they are. Surfing crosses age barriers and has an incredible community. I can be in the water right next to the best surfer in the world, and this has actually happened to me. Very few sports give you that kind of opportunity.

Q: You mentioned that you collect books.

A: I love books. I have a collection of 1,383 books about surfing. It's hard to imagine, but there are fiction, non-fiction and all kinds of books that mention surfing. The collection has become a hobby for me.

Q: Where do you draw your inspiration from?

A: From the fact that there are guys older than me out there and still at it. They are in their seventies and eighties and still out there having fun. After all, the best surfer in the water is the one having the most fun.

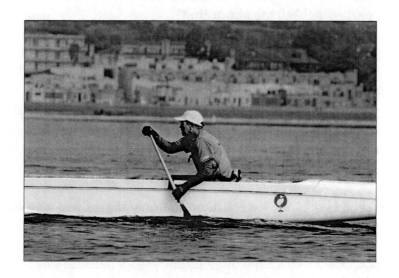

Dave Dyc on the water.

"There's only one captain of the canoe and if you're not him, shut up and paddle."

- Dave Dyc

Innovator Dave Dyc is a 71-year-old outrigger canoe paddler, who splits his time between the shores of Santa Cruz, California and Hilo, Hawaii. He is a retired San Francisco firefighter who enjoyed swimming and surfing while growing up on the California beaches. A firefighter friend of his introduced him to a canoe club about 17 years ago, and Dave loved the solitude of paddling and the workout it gave him.

His friends call him "Lucky," since Dave has had hip, knee and back surgeries; is missing a finger; and has only one eye that he can see out of. Most of these injuries are due to his demanding career as a firefighter. He considers himself lucky to have found an activity that has him out on the ocean nearly every day where he enjoys the vistas while exercising.

Q: With respect to just one of the troubles you've had, you nearly died! Tell me about that!

A: Thirteen years ago I contracted flesh-eating bacteria, which I believe I picked up doing electrical work. I remember reaching around in an attic and I got pricked by a nail or something. I came home and within 24 hours I had a red line up my arm and I almost died. My temperature rose to 107 degrees, I went into shock, and my wife had the priest come in and give me last rights. In the hospital they told me that if I survived, I would lose my arm and probably my feet.

When I woke up a week later, the only thing I had lost was one finger. The only reason I didn't end up worse off is that my lung capacity was good from paddling and swimming. My doctor from that time often tells my story because I was one of his successes. *That experience changed me a whole lot. I quit getting upset at the small stuff.*

Q: I can see why they call you "Lucky," but with all of your surgeries and disabilities what is important to you about working out?

A: Despite these things, I'd like to keep paddling on a regular basis for a long time. At my age, it's not about winning, winning, winning.

Q: What can you tell me about your training?

A: I don't do much cross training. I've had hip and knee surgery, so I'm not a great walker or runner. I'm lucky to spend a lot of time on the water; I put in 30-to-35 miles a week and I'm on the water daily. It's time on the water that helps me the most. I also use a GPS so that I can easily track where I am, and I use a heart rate monitor. These are very important for my training. The GPS gives me my boat speed and rowing time, and the heart rate monitor helps me hit my target workout zone.

Q: What about your sport motivates you?

A: I try to improve a little bit each time I go out paddling. The great thing about paddling is that every day is a new sightseeing adventure. I often listen to music when I paddle and watch the beautiful scenery.

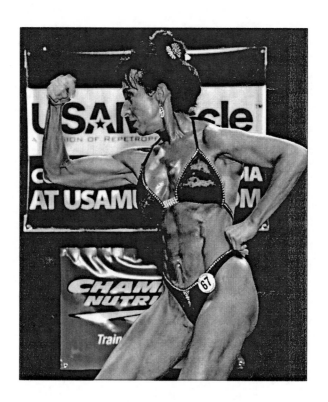

Maria Riquet showing strong.

"I visualize what I want to achieve."
- Maria Riquet

Innovator Maria Riquet is a 57-year-old bodybuilder. Originally from Brazil, where she danced ballet and played tennis when she was young, she came to the United States to get a college education. When she moved to Albuquerque, New Mexico, Maria took up running and ran for many years, although not competitively.

She was motivated to stay in shape and look good, so when she was raising her children, she would run early in the morning before her husband left for work. When her kids got older, she discovered cycling and became a competitive masters cyclist, winning Florida state championships.

In 2003, Maria had a terrible cycling accident. The driver of a car hit her cycling group head-on, and this left her fighting for her life. She had many broken bones, but the worst was her shinbone, which was broken in 30 pieces.

From her hospital bed, Maria remembered that while raising her sons, she used to watch a bodybuilding show on ESPN. Memories of that show inspired her to visualize being able to exercise again. While the doctors were telling her that she would never be able to do hard work with her legs, Maria was envisioning strengthening and honing her body to that of a bodybuilder. Three years after the accident, she competed in her first bodybuilding competition and even placed fourth. A year later, she won that same competition.

Maria works out with a bunch of very strong male bodybuilders, who refer to her as "The Beast," because she works out so hard. No doubt the doctors who put Maria back together would be shocked to see her leg press 365 pounds.

Q: How has that horrifying cycling accident affected your life?

A: That day, before I had my bike accident, I got my gear pouch, my jersey, my keys, hopped on the bike, and was set for a great ride, never thinking that my life would be forever changed. I loved that bike so much that I used to call it my husband.

Having recovered from the accident, I see it as my duty to inspire others and convey to them that anything is possible. If I could take my body from where it was after the accident, to where it is today, then others can make transformations in their lives. I am currently helping a woman lose some weight and get in shape, who is new to working out. She is very grateful to be making such a big transition. I am happy that I can inspire her to change her life.

Q: What's it like to be a bodybuilder at age 57 and how are you so successful?

A: To tell you the truth, no 57-year-old woman is body building at the level that I am. Most don't workout as hard as I do. I honestly don't know if I'm physically stronger, or if it's my powerful will that sets me apart. I visualize what I want to achieve, and constantly tell myself that if I want to reach my goal I need to do my workouts and hold to my diet. For example, when I'm preparing for a big competition, to burn off fat I have to walk for an hour every day before I workout. I have to tell myself that this is what I need to do if I want to win.

Q: What was the best advice you were ever given?

A: My wisdom came from my dad and my mom. My dad used to wake up every morning and do Tai Chi. He would only eat what was necessary; he never ate until he was full. At an early age I learned discipline and the importance of physical exercise. I paid attention to what I ate. My mom also used to tell me never to walk with my chin down, and to always feel good and be happy. I have taught my kids similar lessons.

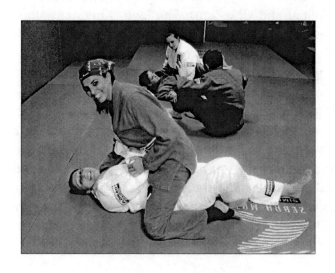

Cheryl Ragsdale working the mat.

"Yes or no, but never maybe."
- Cheryl Ragsdale

While writing my book, I put together a slide show with pictures of the athletes I interviewed. Each had the athlete's name, age, and location, as well as a quote from the interview. The most common reaction when Bloomer Cheryl Ragsdale's slide emerged was, "She can't be over-50." She most certainly is, and a great example of the magic of leading an active life and having a sense of fun. Cheryl is an amazingly youthful 51-year-old boxer and martial arts artist who lives in Boston, Massachusetts.

At age 46, she started working out, taking aerobics classes, and lifting weights. She enjoyed working out this way, but her life was changed one day when at her gym, her future boxing trainer told her that she had a long reach. Cheryl didn't understand, so she asked him what he meant. He said, "Hold out your arm. Look how long your arm is." He went on to explain that he operated a boxing gym in town. He invited her to visit, and the first time she tried boxing she lit up. A year ago, Cheryl took up Brazilian Jujitsu and kickboxing. She loves how martial arts bring out the warrior in her, and it had another surprising effect.

Q: Being a woman in a boxing gym must be an interesting experience. Tell me about it.

A: The gym where I first trained is a very masculine place. I was one of the few women who worked out there. I began wondering how I fit into that environment. The men there, and some were really tough guys, did treat me differently. I noticed that when a new guy would come into the gym, they'd look at me trying to figure out how I fit in. The other guys would non-verbally tell them that it was my place too, and not to mess with me.

I started to realize that I was different and that was okay. I didn't need to fit in with the guys. I said to myself, "Wow, I can be a complete girl here," which is different from how I operated in the rest of the world. This had the unexpected affect of making me gentler than before I started martial arts.

Q: You sound excited. What about your sport motivates you?

A: I fell in love with martial arts. I just *Love It!* I don't think I'd still be going to the gym often if I hadn't discovered boxing. Aerobics classes were nice, but they didn't catch my attention the way martial arts have.

Q: What are you most proud of in boxing?

A: I don't spar or fight, so what I'm most proud of is that I was given a nickname. I'm "The First Lady of FloMAC." FloMAC is the name of my gym. I was the first woman to sign up and I'm currently the highest-level woman martial artist in our gym. I am a white belt, with four (yay!) stripes. FloMAC has been open for about a year, and I intend to be the first female black belt trained by them.

Q: What would be your ultimate achievement?

A: Getting that black belt, and along the way, I'd love to knit the skills of boxing, Jiujitsu, and kickboxing together, and actually engage in fun sparring. That would be so cool. I would love to have the stamina to last a full five-minute round, as well as have the required ability to relax and concentrate.

Q: Do you have a saying or motto that you live your life by?

A: Accept "yes" or "no," but never "maybe." I like to be clear about things. If it's yes, it's yes. If it's no, it's no. Maybe is a holding pattern like being in quicksand, and it holds people back.

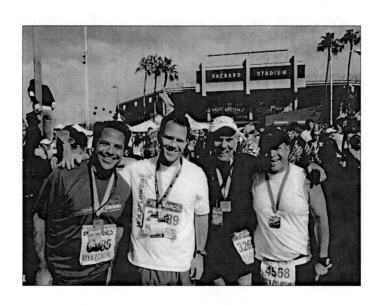

Merrill Schwartz (second from right) with
three of his sons.

"Be committed and follow through."
- Merrill Schwartz

Bloomer Merrill Schwartz is a 67-year-old triathlete, who lives and practices law in San Francisco, California. Merrill started cycling when he was in his thirties in an effort to lose weight. He found it much easier to increase his activity level rather than eat less, because he really likes to eat.

With four young boys in the family and a busy law practice, Merrill picked up running so that he could get a higher intensity workout in a shorter amount of time. About 17 years ago, his son Brian was volunteering at a triathlon, and Merrill figured that he cycled and ran, so why not do a triathlon? He is very happy with the diversity that triathlon training offers.

Merrill was green long before it was fashionable. He has been cycling to work for over 40 years. He is as committed to cycling to work as he is to his family and his clients. Each day he rides his folding bike three miles to the train, lifts it onto the train, and then rides four miles from the train station to his office.

Q: What is your biggest accomplishment in your sports?
A: Having run with each of my four sons when they did their first marathon. That meant a lot to me.

Q: It must have been a challenge being an attorney, raising a large family, and training. What's your biggest challenge now?
A: I don't have enough time to do my work and the activities I love, to the extent that I would like to. That's the biggest challenge, getting everything I want and need to do, done in the day. I try to manage it by setting aside time for my sports activities, just like I do for a client appointment or a court appearance.

Q: As an over-50 athlete, what do you consider to be the keys to you success?

A: I think at my age, it is consistency and continuing without taking a long break except for injuries. Even when I'm injured, I cross train. It takes a lot longer now for me to get back into shape if I let myself get out of shape. Fortunately, I live in San Francisco where it's neither too hot nor too cold, and I can train all year round.

Q: As you've become older, how do you stay motivated?

A: I was complaining to an ex-football player friend of mine about how I get discouraged because I'm no longer able to keep up with the front of the pack – or even the middle of the pack. He said, "You don't always have to be the best. Mentally go out there and do your best and don't expect to be king of the hill anymore. We're too old to be the king of the hill." This was significant for me, and I realized that I need to be able to mentally get through the discouragement, and believe that I don't have to be the best anymore.

Q: Where does your inspiration come from?

A: I get inspired by younger people. Part of the reason I think we compete is because we have the younger group pushing us. The people who go out there to look good, act well and try hard, inspire me.

***

What Can You Do with Your Own Performance-to-Lifestyle Transition?

It's time to apply the lessons in this chapter to your situation. Move yourself further along to a strong, healthy life. From what you've read, you'll know if you are an Innovator, Bloomer, or Groover. Of course, becoming a Groover isn't easy. A person has to start at a young age and must have especially good fortune, and a very unique mind-set. It's certainly easier to become an Innovator or Bloomer, and that's what most of us are.

Whatever their approach to exercise or sports, the 50 athletes over 50 that I interviewed are great role models for successful Performance-to-Lifestyle Transitions. You can learn from their techniques and apply them as you work toward developing a sustained active lifestyle.

The following written *Do It!* exercises are designed to help you with your own transition. They are meant to stimulate your interest in the four joys: joy of good health, joy of movement, joy of achievement, and the joy of association. They are designed to put you on the path to becoming an Innovator or a Bloomer.

Do It! Exercises
Performance-to-Lifestyle

- Be open to trying new sports or activities. Doing so affords new challenges and a renewed sense of accomplishment. New activities also provide new people to socialize with.

o Is there a particular sport or physical activity that you are curious about, but haven't pursued yet? Maybe one that a friend or relative currently does? If so, what is it?

o What can you do in the next week to find out more about this activity?

If this activity feels like something you want to do, commit to take the action that you listed above in the next week. If after you do that you're still interested, then follow your curiosity.

- Find ways to change your definition of accomplishment by switching to another sport.

  o Is there a twist that you can put in your current sport or activity? Some examples are to switch from aerobics to kick boxing, from cycling road races to time trials. You can run longer or shorter events; or take up duathlons or triathlons to keep running, cycling or swimming interesting.

  o List one or two twists that you want to try out.

  o What action can you take in the next week to explore how you would go about implementing one of the twists you listed?

If a twist feels like something you want to do, commit to take the action you listed in the next week. If you're still are interested, then follow your curiosity.

- Transform your workouts into an adventure that can be more interesting and fun.

Make your exercise more inviting. Adventures can be large or small. Would it be appealing to go to a different gym or walk on a different trail? Would ice skating be an enjoyable change of pace? Maybe you can practice your sport in a new location that seems exciting or interesting. For example, is there a race in Hawaii or Europe that looks like fun? List new opportunities or locations that could enhance your workout.

In the next week, explore whether these hold an adventure that you want to act on; an adventure with which you can merge an exercise goal with a fun experience.

- Develop a community.

If you don't have a strong community of active people to interact with regularly, you can develop one or find one. You can ask friends to join you in your sport; or ask about existing clubs at running stores, cycling shops, or other sports-related businesses. You can also try searching for groups on the Internet using websites like meetup.com and active.com which list thousands of clubs and events all over the United States.

o What action can you take in the next week toward connecting with or developing a community of active people?

If this feels like something that would be helpful, make a commitment to yourself to take the action that you listed in the next week.

You've learned about the Performance-to-Lifestyle Transition, its phases, and how it can be more easily mastered with motivation from the four joys. Different types of athletes and their approach to remaining active were described, and you probably know which type you are.

Now, to understand the transition from a performance focus to a lifestyle focus even better, we'll take a deeper look at the three key phases of the Performance-to-Lifestyle Transition: *Dream It*, *Love It* and *Live It*. Although over-age-50 athletes work with all of these phases, there will be interviews of those who used one particular phase to their best advantage. We'll start off with *Dream It*, the first phase, which allows us to begin imagining participating in a sport or in regular exercise.

Chapter 3: Dream It

"Far away there in the sunshine are my highest aspirations. I may not reach them, but I can look at them and see their beauty, believe in them, and try to follow where they lead."

-Louisa May Alcott

All of the 50 over-50 athletes that I interviewed have the ability to envision, or dream about, doing something out of the ordinary. This plays an important part in having a sustained active life. The process of imagining something that we want is not a secret. All it takes is the confidence to know that your use of mental imagery is powerful.

To create success, we can go over and over our dream goal in our minds. We can visualize what it took others to gain the success that we want. We can practice seeing ourselves achieve similar success. We can map a detailed plan in our minds to be clear about what steps we need to take to achieve our dream. Mapping a detailed plan on paper is yet another way to bring positive results. We can share our dream and enlist the support of family members and good friends. And when we finally realize our dream, we can more confidently share this envisioning process with others who need a boost.

I observed that while all the athletes use the *Dream It* concept to some extent, they do so in three different ways and in varying degrees. A few athletes have goals that are extraordinarily challenging, such as setting a world record, winning national or world championships, or performing incredible feats. Some see themselves as able to perform at remarkably high levels in their sport, despite their ages. Others envision taking up completely new activities later in life; at an age most of us would not consider. I will refer to these three variants as *Dream It—Achievement*, *Dream It—Longevity*, and *Dream It—Possibilities*.

Dream It—Achievement athletes are the rarest of dreamers, as they have managed to hang onto the characteristics of high performance that tends to fade with age. To talk with them is to marvel at how driven they are, despite the physical challenges they face in training as hard as they do. Achievement-oriented athletes tend to get most of their motivation from the joy of accomplishment.

As examples of this type of athlete, I offer interviews with Sandy Scott and Helen Geoffrion. Both have set goals at the national or world championship levels in their age groups. Their trainings are planned around key competitive events that are stepping stones along the way to their ultimate goals. This past year, Sandy was Florida state cycling champion in the 20K time trial, while Helen placed third in the World Triathlon Championships.

Dream It—Longevity athletes, while being aware of the challenges older athletes face, can't envision a life without physical activity. To talk with longevity-led dreamers is to know the timeless joy of practicing their sport. They see themselves leading active lives well into the future.

Examples of these athletes are Jerry Smartt, Katy Okuyama and Gale Bernhardt. Jerry, Katy and Gale envision themselves doing their sport when they are beyond ages 90- to 100-years old.

Jerry is a 77-year-old distance runner who wants to be racing at 100 years of age. Katy is a 53-year-old surfer, who has been surfing since age 16, and hopes to be surfing when she is 90. At 50 years old, Gale is an endurance athlete who is currently focused on the Leadville 100-mile mountain bike race in Leadville, Colorado. In that race, she is two-time champion in her age group. Gale told me that she wants to be competing when she is 100 years old. Wouldn't it be cool to do the Leadville 100 at 100 years old?!

Dream It—Possibilities dreamers are an inspiration to those who have not yet found their exercise or sports passion. They embody the explorer in all of us that, once unleashed, can change our lives forever.

Carol Jean Vosburgh and Terry Peterson are Possibilities examples. Carol Jean took up running in her forties, and has gone on to compete at a high level in running, cycling, and triathlons. At the age of 49, Terry realized that he was gaining unwanted weight. So he picked up mountain unicycling, and has developed his skill, strength, and endurance to an amazing degree.

Regardless of their specific type of *Dream It*, these athletes all demonstrate the ability to see beyond conventional wisdom. They maintain a childlike outlook that enables them to envision themselves doing things far from ordinary. Each, in different ways, can inspire us to visualize ourselves as the strong, healthy people we wish to be. Enjoy the following interviews, keeping their ability to *Dream It* in mind as you read their inspiring stories.

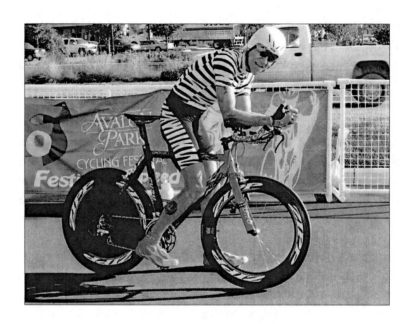

Sandy Scott looking fast!

"Victory belongs to an antagonist who knows how to suffer one quarter hour longer."

- Sandy Scott

Sandy Scott is a colorful 69-year-old elite cyclist who lives in Seminole, Florida. He has managed to pack so much into his life, that its density approaches that of a black hole. I almost felt a gravitational pull when listening to his stories. Sandy had a varied professional career, and at one time or another was a police officer, a military man, a commercial airline pilot, a corporate sales executive, and an entrepreneur. Of all these, Sandy loved the 25 years he spent as an airline pilot the most, and because of this, says he would have done this work for free.

Sandy also has an impressive array of other interests including chess, collections of all kinds, amateur radio, playing drums, martial arts, bass fishing, shooting, and photography. Added to that is skydiving, high-fidelity audio, logic puzzles, motorcycling, electronics, running, tennis, golf, and of course, cycling.

A competitive athlete for most of his life, Sandy won national masters titles in track and cross-country in his late thirties and early forties. He started cycling at age 64 when his now fiancée Rosie, a competitive cyclist in her own right, dropped by his house one day. She told him that she had two bikes and a picnic lunch, and that they were going for a ten-mile ride. Sandy had a blast that day and bought a bike the next week. He found that he had a talent for cycling and within nine months of that first ride, he went under the state record for the 5K time trial. He also turned in the fastest 10K time trial time of the day, out of more than 100 racers in various age groups at a Senior Games event.

Days before I interviewed him, Sandy won the Florida state United States Cycling 20K time trial title, breaking the record he set two years ago by 18 seconds. This is especially astonishing given that at age 65 he had a shocking cycling accident that resulted in a fracture of his C1 vertebra, which is often fatal.

Sandy's dream is to win four gold medals at the 2011 Senior Games in Houston, Texas. He also wishes that all people can get to understand that growing older as an athlete can be a fantastic experience, but it takes work. His advice? Lift weights, eat right, get aerobic exercise, have good relationships, have goals, exercise your mind, have a positive outlook, and get regular medical checkups. This may seem like a lot, but when an athlete is fully engaged in an exercise routine or sport, many of these suggestions become an automatic part of life. But Sandy's keen inner drive to win is another thing.

Q: You are incredibly driven, so what keeps you motivated?

A: The keys are my consistency, having a plan, executing the plan, and being so competitive that I would die rather than lose. Plus, I desperately want to win at everything, and I only want to compete against people who really want to beat me with all their heart. I look around for the most exciting events with the most competition. In one instance I was told that the current national time trial champion would be at an event. I took that as a challenge, signed up, and beat him. I also make it a point to race all of the championship events that are within a reasonable driving distance from where I live.

Next year, I'll be in the 70-year-old age group, and it's almost frustrating for me because at the moment, I just don't have competition in that age group. For example, at the recently completed USCF Florida state 20K time trial championships, the closest time to mine in the 70+ year-old age group was six minutes and ten seconds slower than mine. I just may register in a younger age group so I can have some competition. All the state records would be fairly easy to beat.

Q: You are in awesome condition and are very successful. What's the trick?

A: When I started working at the airline company in my twenties, I was in terrible shape. As a new pilot, I noticed that in the lounge there were a number of obituaries for pilots who were typically around 62-years-old. I found that from an actuarial standpoint, pilots tend to die shortly after retirement. I told myself that would not happen to me. I joined the gym, started lifting weights and never stopped.

I also have great genetics. I have these freaky extra-long lungs, and if I don't tell an x-ray technician that I have them, I'll have to have the x-rays taken again.

Q: You train very hard, so what can you share about your training?

A: I have a plan, I know exactly what I'm going to do, and I do it. I plan for two peaks a year. One peak is for the recent state championships, and the other is for the state Senior Games in December. Every single day I know exactly what my mission is and I execute it. If I wake up and don't feel like doing my intervals, or if it's raining, I make myself do the planned ride anyway. I hope my competitors look outside at the rain and decide to wait until tomorrow. I've only missed one day of riding in a year and a half, and that was due to having a surgery. My doctor wanted me to take off two weeks and I told him I'd give him one day.

Q: Do you have a saying or motto that you like?

A: "Victory belongs to an antagonist who knows how to suffer one quarter hour longer." I was in this race in Ocala, Florida, and this guy in the race was attacking all the hills. I was thinking to myself that I was dying, but just kept hanging on. The guy ended up puking his brains out, and I passed him and won. Never, ever give up.

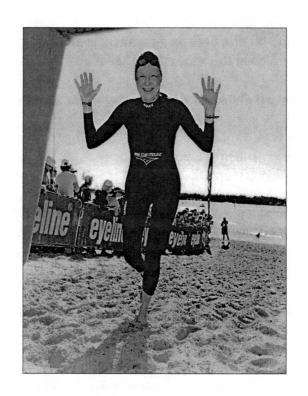

Helen Geoffrion just out of the water.

"Workout less to improve."
- Helen Geoffrion

Helen Geoffrion is a 70-year-old triathlete who lives in Santa Monica, California, and attended a private girl's school in Columbus, Ohio, where she played every sport they offered. This list included tennis, soccer, softball, field hockey, basketball, swimming, and badminton. Helen was recognized as Best Athlete in her high school graduating class. In 2000, she was elected to the Columbus School for Girl's Athletic Hall of Fame for being a great athlete while in school, and because she was one of the first female triathletes in the United States in the 45-year-old age group in the mid-1980s.

Several times, Helen was selected for the USA World Triathlon Team that went to the World Triathlon Championships. While on this team, she traveled to Germany, Switzerland, Australia, New Zealand, and places in the United States. She is often ranked in the top 10 for 14 of the 17 events in USA Masters Swimming.

She started doing triathlons because she enjoys swimming so much. In the mid-1980s, she saw people training for and doing triathlons and thought it looked like fun. She completed an Olympic-length triathlon in her first outing and enjoyed it, despite it being very difficult for her. When Helen called her daughter to tell her that she had done her first triathlon, she was surprised to hear that her daughter had done *her* first triathlon the same weekend!

Helen definitely got the bug and has competed at national and world championship levels in swimming and triathlons ever since. Oddly enough, she told me that while working with her coach Gale Bernhardt, she dropped her training from more than 20 hours per week to 10 hours per week, and has seen great results.

Q: **You found that you were able to *improve* by working out less? Tell me more about that!**

A: I give my coach Gale all the credit. She got me balanced. She and I had to wrestle with it a little bit, though. She had to convince me to spend less time swimming. I love to swim, but I was tiring myself out, so I couldn't train my cycling or running properly. Gale was also very patient with me in my cycling; it took me a long time to learn to spin.

Q: **Is there anything specific you attribute your sustained success to?**

A: I understand now that my key is balance in training; if you do mostly one type of training, your body will break down. I think that because I swim, cycle, and run, my muscles and tendons don't get as worn, and they have been fine. Doing various training routines also keeps it more interesting. I used to swim every day and it can get old. I would go to the pool and have my face in the water for two hours. My trainer has me doing weights as well as cycling, swimming and running, and I've seen tremendous improvement since I started working with Gale.

I'm also a high-energy person. I can clean the house all afternoon and then empty the pond of water. I run circles around my husband! I just have an awful lot of innate energy. I was energetic as a kid and it hasn't subsided. I'm just not moving in the slow lane.

Q: **With all those achievements behind you, is there something else you would like to accomplish?**

A: It would be to climb Mount Everest. It would be hard because I don't like the cold much, nor working out at altitude, but I watch people doing it and it does look like fun.

Q: **What is your biggest challenge?**

A: Cycling. My bike split is always my slowest triathlon split relative to my competitors. In a race I just did, people were ten minutes ahead of me on the bike, but I was 15 minutes ahead of them on the swim, so it was okay. I try to not let it get to me. I don't have much cycling background and I've got long, skinny legs that I think don't help me be a fast cyclist. I have gotten a lot faster in recent years.

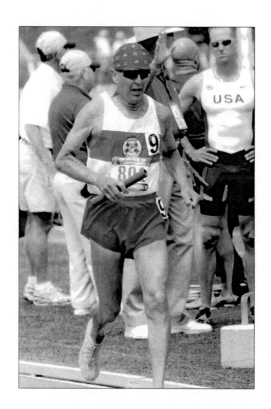

Jerry Smartt on the track.

"It's no hill for a climber, young fellow."
- Jerry Smartt

Jerry Smartt is a 77-year-old runner, who lives in Warsaw, Missouri, and has been running for 62 years. A retired English teacher, Jerry has loved footraces his whole life. He got his start playing tag and hide-and-go-seek when he was a child. His talents went untapped until he was a senior in high school, and some friends of his who were on the track team told the team coach that Jerry was one fast cat. Jerry joined the team, and with perseverance went on to win many races.

In 1952, he joined the Air Force and had great success as a runner. He even qualified as an alternate for the 1956 Olympics in Melbourne, Australia.

Jerry continues to run and compete at the national level because he still loves a footrace, and because he feels it has given him the great health he currently enjoys. He keeps a scrapbook with media clippings from his running career. It currently weighs 40 pounds and in it he has eight aliases. His favorite alias is from a Finnish newspaper, in which he is named "Josef Smargg."

Q: Being alternate on the Olympic team is a huge accomplishment, so do you consider that your greatest achievement?
A: Running races when I hit 100 years old would be my ultimate achievement. I have wonderful health and I don't know how long it will last, but I plan on still running when I'm 100. If something happens that I can't run, I'll walk. I saw an overweight young gal and she was walking three miles. I congratulated her and told her she needs to think about working up to walking three or four hours. She looked at me like I had just landed from outer space. Walking is great exercise, but most walkers don't walk far enough to really get a workout.

Q: Given that you've been at it for 62 years, racing at 100 doesn't sound unreasonable. How have you stayed with it

for so long?

A: Of all the guys from the 1956 and 1958 national teams, I'm the only one who is still competing. The others may be doing things to stay fit, but they are not in the big meets, like nationals. Many of these guys gave up running in their thirties and gained weight. My mindset is what differentiates me from the guys who stopped running. I made up my mind a long time ago that I'm never going to voluntarily stop running. Running keeps me healthy and it's no longer about the trophies. I'm still having fun.

Q: Is there anything specific you do in training that you feel is a key to your success?

A: I do resistance training; things that are really difficult. For example, I have an ATV tire with a rope tied to it, with the other end tied to an old shirt. I tie the shirt around my waist and run 100-yard sprints 30 times, with short rests. Sometimes I'll do this while pushing a shopping cart full of concrete blocks. It looks kind of funny, but I gain strength and lung power. I also simulate altitude by holding my breath while I'm running. I'll hold my breath for a couple hundred yards, which forces my body to produce more red blood cells, like I'm training at altitude. I've been doing that for a long time.

Q: What are your goals and how do you set them?

A: In the past, my goals were to be ready to run nationals, beat a certain time, or to complete a tough workout. I used to run unbelievable workouts, like 40 times a quarter mile, or four times a mile in four minutes and forty seconds.

My goal now is to stay healthy and pace everything, so tomorrow I can be doing again what I do today. I still do races and I use those to stay motivated.

Q: Do you have any challenges?

A: My biggest challenge is staying healthy. I don't train as hard as I'd like to train because I've learned that if I train too hard,

I will get hurt. I run twice a day and my repeat 100- and 200-meter sprints feel rapid, but they are well controlled.

I pace myself and remain aware. I use a stopwatch, wear a GPS to measure my mileage, and I don't knock myself out in workouts. When I was younger I felt bulletproof and ran really hard workouts. I did them because I knew that my competition wasn't, and when I got in a race I knew I was going to perform well.

Q: Is there one particular race that you feel was a breakthrough for you?

A: When I was in the service, I was running well and ran a three-mile race in 15:05, which was an Air Force record. Shortly after that, I ran in an all-star meet with Army, Navy, and some Japanese runners. In the 5K, I looked up at the clock and saw my time at three miles was under 15 minutes, and I thought to myself that maybe I had something going. Fifteen minutes for three miles at the time was a big deal.

That spring, at the Olympic trials, there were some 35 guys in the 10K race and all the elites from the 1952 Olympics were there. I was not well known, but they had heard about my good times in the prior weeks. At one point in the race, I was in about 20th place when I started passing people. I passed one guy and he said, "Go on Jerry." I then passed another guy, and he said, "Go Jerry," and another and another. These were the former elite runners and they were cheering me on. I ended up in 4th place. I often think that if I knew these guys a little better, I may have finished even higher.

Q: Do you have a saying or motto that you live your life by?

A: When I was on a team being coached by the great hurdler Johnny Morris, we would have to drag this metal mesh around the track to flatten out the cinders. We would complain about that or about how hard a workout was, and Johnny would look at us and say, "No hill for a climber, young fellow." He always impressed on us that, whatever the difficulty, we could overcome it. When I'm at races, I like to yell to the runners, "Run like the wind." I have that on my medic alert bracelet along with my identification.

***

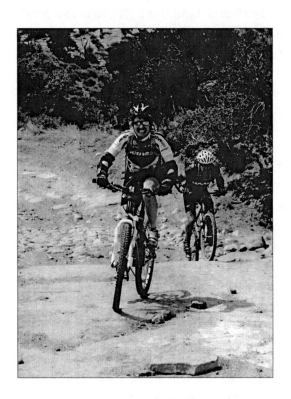

Gale Bernhardt, enjoying the climb.

"When people ask me what I'm training for, I tell them that I'm training for life, because it requires tremendous endurance."

- Gale Bernhardt

Fifty-year-old Gale Bernhardt is a self-proclaimed endurance sport junkie, who lives in Loveland, Colorado. An engineer, Gale left her job at a major corporation over a decade ago to follow her dream and become a coach. She has participated in many sports over the past 40 years including triathlons, swimming, cycling, trail running, and skiing. Gale loves helping people achieve their goals. Her personal sports focus over the past five years has been the 100-mile "Leadville 100" mountain bike race in Leadville, Colorado. To officially complete the race, you need to finish the course in less than 12 hours.

In her first Leadville 100, Gale approached the finish line with crowds lining the street and a Tour-de-France-like finish as she crossed the line at 11:59.55 – a mere five seconds from the cut-off time. That experience hooked Gale on this race, and earned her the prestigious Last Ass over the Pass Trophy, which is one of her most treasured possessions. In 2008 and 2009, she won the Leadville 100 in her age group. She looks forward to pedaling strong, and placing well in the 2010 race.

Gale's interview is one of a handful that I conducted in person, and when I first met her, I understood why she is a great coach. Her enthusiasm shines in her eyes and her positive attitude is contagious.

Q: You have done so much. What would be your ultimate achievement?
A: I want to still be doing endurance events when I'm 100 years old.

Q: You have been so consistently successful in a number of endurance sports. How do you do it?

A: For me, consistency itself trumps everything. I keep a regular routine and I don't take big blocks of time off.

Q: **I hear that you like fun and adventure. How do they fit in?**

A: I do whatever sounds fun, and sometimes I go out looking for adventures that I'm not sure I can do. I love the adventure of thinking I can do something, but not really being sure of it.

Q: **Where do you draw your inspiration from?**

A: Everyone, everywhere around me. 99 percent of the people I talk to have had positive and inspiring stories, in which they overcame something, achieved something, or had some great adventure.

Q: **Anything else you'd like to share?**

A: People can do anything they want to do. We just need to be able to pick the goal and make the appropriate sacrifices. It's risky, because you might not succeed, but you just might.

***

Katy Okuyama having fun.

"Don't give up. Just keep plugging at it and you'll get it."

- Katy Okuyama

Katy Okuyama is a 53-year-old surfer who lives in Honolulu, Hawaii, and has passion for food as well as surfing. Her grandfather and father were both grocers, and Katy has carried on their love of good food by working as a natural and organic food broker.

While surfing doesn't go as far back as her family's love of food, Katy has been surfing since she was 16 years old. Her older sister and older brother both surfed, and Katy took over her brother's surfboard when he went away to college. She was immediately taken with the sport. She tried to give up surfing in college, so that she could focus on her studies, but the ocean's call got to her and she returned to surfing. She loves the ocean and feels that its ionic effects help her stay energized. Katy hopes to be surfing when she reaches 90.

Q: You've been surfing since you were 16, so how do you stay motivated with one sport for so long?

A: I am drawn to the ocean. I love getting in the water and feeling good. I read that that the ocean has positive ions and your body has negative ions, so when you go into the ocean, the positive and negative ions interact and make you feel good. This is my experience, and I will always live by the ocean.

Q: What about surfing are you most proud of?

A: I've been surfing for 37 years now. I'm 53-years-old and still surfing. My daughter is 28, and I've been surfing longer than she's been on this earth. There are a lot of people who stop being active when they get older, but I feel that life is too short to do that. Anything can happen, and I've had close friends become ill, so I try not to waste any days. So to be healthy, for me, is to be able to go to the ocean to surf. If not surfing, go swimming, go body boarding or even go for walk on the beach. I always look forward to it. It feels too good to pass up!

Q: You feel intensely about food as well as about surfing. Do you see any parallels?

A: I've seen people come and go in both surfing and the food business. In order to stick with either for a long period of time you need to have great passion. Passion can give you incredible drive and focus, and allows you to keep at it.

Q: What advice would you give to people just getting started in a sport or exercise program?

A: Don't give up. Just keep plugging at it and you'll get it.

***

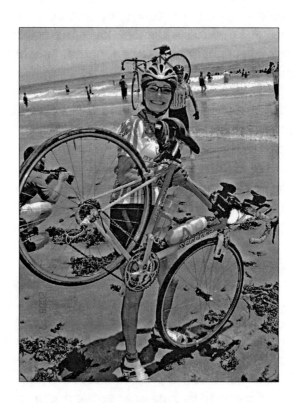

Carol Jean Vosburgh starting a grand adventure.

"Live passionately with no regrets."
- Carol Jean Vosburgh

Carol Jean Vosburgh is a 63-year-old cyclist who lives in Treasure Island, Florida, and recently retired from working as a registered nurse. Carol Jean was a late starter and didn't take up any sort of sport until she was nearing her 40th birthday. As a single parent of three, she was looking for stress relief and had a choice to make. She could either join the crowd at work that went out drinking after hours, or she could join the group of people who ran at lunch time. She chose running.

While running was hard for her at first, she soon found herself able to run farther and farther. At 41, Carol Jean entered her first running race, a Thanksgiving Day "Turkey Trot," and won in her age group. She was thrilled to have gone from never having competed in any sporting event, to having won her very first race. She loved competing and being around her healthy running friends – especially given the pain, suffering, and death she saw at work. She moved on to doing triathlons and has come to appreciate the diversity that triathlon training offers. Eventually, Carol Jean qualified for the Kona Ironman.

When she was 62, Carol Jean and her husband joined a group of bicyclists to ride the 4,000 miles from the San Francisco bay to the New Hampshire shore. As she does nothing on a small scale, she and her companions completed the ride in 52 days.

A strong woman, she has worked through many setbacks including open heart surgery at the age of 52. After that, Carol Jean first thought that she might never run again. Nonetheless, she is now training to win four or more gold medals in cycling, running, and the triathlon at the 2011 Senior Games in Houston, Texas.

Q: Tell me more about your ride across the country and the breakthrough you had?

A: I had a breakthrough on the cross-country bicycle ride when I stretched way out of my comfort zone. My husband and I signed up with a group that was riding from California to New Hampshire. We trained hard for the six months leading up to the ride, and about a week before the ride I tried to back out. It hit me that I didn't like riding downhill and we had many passes to ride over. If they had given me my money back, I would have backed out.

I didn't have confidence in myself. We started the ride by dipping one wheel in the Pacific Ocean and off we went. After one week, I had decided the ride was really fun and that I was probably one of the stronger riders. We ended the ride by dipping our wheel in the Atlantic Ocean and the vision of that is what kept me going mile after mile.

Q: What are the key aspects of your training?
A: Moderation and consistency. I bike three days a week, run three days a week, and lift weights three days a week. I do this consistently and I think this is the reason I've been able to continue doing what I do. I'm also a firm believer in stretching, because as we age we get less flexible and we really need to stretch. I'm also a big believer in lifting weights. You need upper body strength, even for running and cycling.

Q: What is the biggest challenge you face?
A: Keeping my life balanced. I have a hard time taking a day off. I could train all day long because I *Love It*. I just think it's fun and I just *Love It* out there. It is my personality to be that way, so the hardest thing for me is keeping my life in balance. I have had numerous injuries and it's those times that teach me to listen to my body. I manage this challenge by filling my life with other things like working with my church, going to movies, and reading.

Q: How else do you keep your sport balanced in your life?
A: I don't set as aggressive goals as I used to, which also makes

it more fun. I want to keep my church work, husband, kids, and grandkids all in balance. My big goal is winning gold medals at the 2011 Senior Games. That's the long-term goal, but next year I'll start doing a lot of different events just to get ready for 2011. I will start with little steps and take an incremental approach. I do well by racing myself into shape over a longer period of time, rather than building to a peak quickly.

Q: To what do you attribute the tremendous athletic success you are having in your sixties?

A: One thing is that I started later, so I wasn't burned out like many others who started when they were younger. I've met a lot of people who were really active in sports when they were younger, but got burned out. I never did anything before I was almost 40, so I was the newbie who had lots of energy. When I was young, girls didn't do any sports for the most part. There wasn't much opportunity back then, prior to Title IX legislation. I got married at 17 and by the time I was 23, I had three kids. My exercise was running after my kids. When I was introduced to running and found out that I had natural ability, you can imagine how much pent up energy I had.

Q: What was the best advice you were ever given?

A: When the going gets tough, the tough get going. Other good advice is to live passionately with no regrets. It is my mantra that I'm always repeating to myself.

Q: Anything else you'd like to share?

A: *I think it's really important that we give back and inspire other people. Sports have given me so much, and it's very important to mentor and help others. When you help someone else, they win and you win doubly. I've told many people that getting into running saved my life. I was at a very low period in my life when I found running and it pulled me up and gave me a positive focus.*

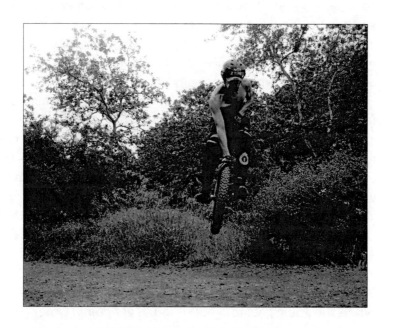

Terry Peterson dreaming big air.

"Life is very much like mountain unicycling. It's not about avoiding the obstacles, but meeting them head-on and overcoming them."

- Terry Peterson

Terry Peterson is a 53-year-old mountain unicyclist from Redondo Beach, California, and he has what I'll call a "nuclear" personality. His energy and passion for MUni, as it's called, is palpable, even over the phone. Terry participated in running and golf over the years, but only came to Mountain Unicycling (MUni) about three and a half years ago. He found that in his late forties he had gained weight, had high cholesterol, and got winded very easily. Tuning and servicing pianos at his business had him fairly sedentary during much of his workday. Running bothered his knees, bicycling seemed boring, swimming was inconvenient, and he was searching for what to do.

Bingo, he stumbled on the website unicycle.com, and was amazed to see how far the advances in unicycles had come since he last rode on in his teens. Fast forward to today, Terry is a sponsored and extremely accomplished MUni rider. MUni has become an integral part of his life, and he has extensive footage of his riding on his website, unigeezer.com. Since riding MUni he's lost 31 pounds of fat, gone from a 34" to a 29" waist, and is in the best shape of his life.

Terry has received hundreds of emails and letters from people who see his website, or see an interview with him on radio or TV. A common theme in the letters he receives are writers who thought he was too old to ride, but after seeing his videos, they realized they need to rethink this.

Q: What about your participation in MUni are you most proud of?

A: It's achieving such a high level of skill at my age, and continuing to improve well into my fifties, when so many people my age or younger seem content to sit in front of the TV getting fat and growing old. That's not going to happen with me.

Q: I've seen some of the videos you have on your website, unigeezer.com, and have watched you maneuver tough trails and do incredible jumps on the unicycle. How do you do it?

A: I constantly visualize what I want to do or accomplish. I can achieve probably close to 100 percent of what I see myself doing in my mind's eye. Having the confidence and committing yourself to each task is key to being successful. I go to bed at night visualizing the next line I'm going to ride.

Like a karate guy breaking boards, who doesn't visualize hitting the board, but sees past the board. When I'm visualizing a jump over a gap or a hole, I visualize not just getting to the other side, but beyond the edge.

I ride pretty much every day. During the weekdays I ride before or after work, for one to one-and-a-half hours. On the weekend are the bigger rides where I go farther away, let my hair down, scout out other places, and spend hours out there.

Q: Is there any particular thing you'd like to achieve in MUni?

A: I want to ride MUni at a high level well into my eighties. To me that would be the most awesome thing. Another thing I'd like to do is get on Letterman's, Conan's, or Leno's show. Not just for myself, but to spread the word to the world that people can do these things at my age. I also want people to know that mountain unicycling is an up-and-coming, legitimate, serious sport, and not something just done by people with frizzy red hair and rubber noses.

Q: Have you experienced a breakthrough, and if so, what led to it?

A: Every day is a breakthrough for me. I live life with gusto and when I go to bed at night, I can't wait to get up the next day.

Not just to ride, but to greet the day, to do the work that I love doing. So that's the breakthrough. Attack every day with love and the passion for life.

Q: What is the best advice you were ever given?
A: No one ever achieves greatness by playing it safe. Sometimes the greatest encouragement one can receive is the discouragement of a nonbeliever.

***

We just saw that athletes in the *Dream It* interviews demonstrate their ability to envision themselves doing something out of the ordinary and use these visions to fuel their active life. The following *Do It!* exercises are designed to make you think about how you currently dream, how you can dream more, and how you can dream in different ways. If right now you cannot fathom an athletic lifestyle, visualizing is the way to start.

Do It! Exercises
Dream It

- What athlete did you most associate with in your ability to *Dream It*?

- o Is there something that they do that you haven't done, but that you would like to do? If so, what is it?

- o What can you do in the next week to understand whether this is something that you should pursue?

o If this feels like something you want to follow up
   on, and then commit to take the action you
   listed above. After you have taken that action, if it
   seems right, continue to pursue it.

- Do you have a *Dream It* goal, and if so what is it?

o If you don't have one, would you like to? If so,
   write down a list of wild, far-out-there aspirations,
   paying no attention to whether they seem realis-
   tic or not. Then sort the list by putting the things
   that excite you the most at the top. Take your top
   goal and start to write down a plan as to when and
   how you will work to achieve it.

- What is the vision you have for yourself at 100 years old?

  o Are you satisfied with this vision?

    o If not, let yourself dream up a new, wild vision of your century-old self and write it down here.

- From the *Do It!* exercises in the previous chapter, is there an activity that you would like to try that you haven't? If so, what's stopping you?

o Is there something you can do to eliminate the thing or things that are stopping you? If so, what can you do in the next week to eliminate what is holding you back?

o If this really seems like something you want to do, then in the next week commit to take the action you listed above.

Through these interviews, we have seen the various ways that some of the over-50 athletes *Dream It*. Dreaming a thing, is the first step towards having it in our lives, and this starts with the confidence to know that using mental imagery is powerful. Athletic dreams that we can envision run the gamut from seeing the simple opportunity to finding the exercise that is right for us, to performing a physical activity at an astounding level.

We found three different *Dream It* approaches, used by over-50 athletes to create a vision and work to make it a reality. *Dream It—Achievement* visualization leads to high performance, despite the physical changes of aging. *Dream It—Longevity* visionaries demonstrate the belief in exercising rigorously at an advanced age. With *Dream It—Possibilities*, the athletes set out to conquer an exercise or sport that they have had no experience with, often later in life when no one expects it. Their examples show us how finding our preferred sport can transform our lives.

Next up, is the *Love It* phase, in which we will see the importance of movement and play in living a strong, healthy life.

Chapter 4: Love It

"In every real man a child is hidden that wants to play."

-Friedrich Nietzsche

I was about two thirds of the way through the 50 interviews, and interviewing one of the athletes. I was saying that it looked like loving a sport is significant in living a strong, healthy life. The interviewee caught me a bit off guard by asking me why this is the case. I had no good answer, just that the information from the interviews showed that this is consistently true. Our exchange launched me on a quest to understand why this is so, as passion seems to play a great role in staying active.

Around this time, I became aware of research done by professors Nikola Medic and Patricia Weir's teams from McMaster University and Canada University of Windsor. Their study examined the motivations of masters athletes, and it was based on surveys of participants in the 2004 Canadian and United States Masters Track and Field Championships. In response to the question "What is the top reason that you maintain your motivation to train?", the most common response was "Enjoyment/ Love of Sport."[1] I could easily agree, since the over-50 athletes I interviewed said that they too, loved their sports. Yet, I felt like there was something missing.

Overweight and Under Motivated

As with many other experiences I've had in doing research for this book, the answer came when I least expected it. I was attending a talk by Dr. John Ratey, professor of psychiatry at Harvard University. In his book *Spark: the Revolutionary New Science of Exercise and the Brain* he explains the neuroscience behind the benefits of exercise. Some points he makes are how exercise prepares the brain to learn, lowers stress, controls hormonal fluctuations, staves off addiction, improves moods and focus, and even reverses some aging effects in the brain.

During his speech, he told us that we have shocking levels of obesity in the United States. Sixty-seven percent of people are overweight and over 30 percent are obese! Worse still, twenty percent of our four year olds are obese. He also informed us of the prevalence of several diseases associated with obesity, including Alzheimer's. Dr. Ratey said that a higher incidence of this disease is seen in obese individuals, and went so far as to refer to Alzheimer's disease as type 3 diabetes. Diabetes is thought, in part, to be managed by keeping a healthy weight through regular physical activity and eating appropriate foods in proper portions.

Dr. Raty also commented that people in today's culture seek convenience, so we don't have much need for physical activity to accomplish daily tasks. By comparison, our ancestors were hunter-gatherers and endurance predators, who covered an average of 14 miles per day. I reminded myself that with the passing of the Industrial Revolution and the advent of the Information Age, the amount of physical exercise the average person now gets is much less – less than one mile per day. The promotion of a high calorie, fast-food mentality combined with a sedentary lifestyle in a high-tech society, makes the need for physical activity among our children even more acute. We wouldn't trade places with a caveman, but clearly, exercise can play a big part in preventing obesity.

Play is Powerful

Dr. Ratey suggested that all children have an innate instinct for active play, but that society both pulls and pushes us away from it as we mature. We are pulled away from play by the busyness that results from the complex demands of work, family, social, and other responsibilities. We are also pushed from engaging in this pleasure by societal norms that value hard work above play.

In our society, working hard to the point of sacrificing personal joy is typically held in high regard, and worn as a badge of courage. In many environments, whether at work or at home, people who make time for fun are seen as slackers. Unfortunately, this attitude instills excessive seriousness and fear in those who would otherwise be playful. Some studies show that employees who enjoy their time at work are more productive. Fear seldom drives healthy behaviors, and our well-being suffers when we yield to these external pressures.

According to Dr. Ratey, nearly all animals play, and active play has a critical role in the development of strength, quickness, and agility. He added that play also helps us to deal with uncertainty and the unexpected. Our bodies actually have mechanisms that make us want to play. There are things called mechanoreceptors that sense the forces exerted by our muscles, and when stimulated give us a pleasurable sensation. We also know that when we exercise hard, wonderful brain chemistry kicks in and gives us the sensation of happiness. Feeling good is a powerful incentive for physical activity.

But most compelling for me was Dr. Ratey's statement that *one of the best ways to activate creativity and playful thinking, is to move our bodies*. After hearing this, I had a revelation. It occurred to me that *the 50 athletes I interviewed have been able to keep their love of play*. By their ability to rouse their childlike urges to visualize playing and to engage in play, it appears that they can regenerate their love for movement and fun. In interviews, they told me that they felt enthusiastic about their workouts, and that the disciplines that went along with a sport seemed more like fun than work.

Now I got it. The promise of play, of fun, keeps athletes coming back for more. Those I interviewed routinely tap their innate instinct to play, which feeds the joy of movement and makes it easier for them to workout regularly and stay with it. The movement in their workouts further stimulates the play instinct, and this connection creates strong motivation to return for the next workout.

A histogram in *Figure 1* (on next page) shows the ages during which the 50 athletes began their first sport, as well as the age they started the exercise that they currently do. On average, they began their first sport at age 15. Some were not active until their forties, but the majority started young. It may be that discovering the love of moving their bodies through sports at an early age, has made it possible for many of these athletes to continue to access their instinct to play. This underscores the importance of instilling a love for physical activity in our youth, as it is more likely they will be active later in life. One way we can do this is by being good role models and taking responsibility for our own active lives. The health of our children could depend on it.

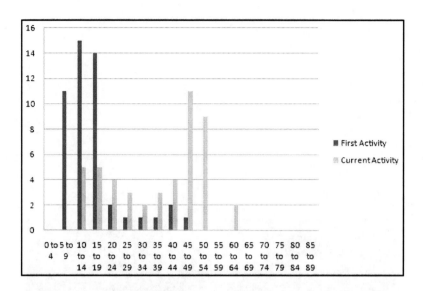

Figure 1: Histogram of the age that 50 over-age-50 athletes be-gan routine exercise or sports, and the age at which they started their current exercise program.

The idea that older athletes who sustain their exercise can connect to childlike playfulness, fits well with the survey results presented in the Performance-to-Lifestyle chapter. Those results showed that play, or movement, was the most important of the four joys in providing motivation. And why not? Movement that gives way to play ignites the body's physical and mental receptors associated with loving a sport or exercise. From an emotional standpoint, movement causes people to banter and to jest. Further, laughter is often a byproduct of the physical action and joy that we experience when we walk with friends, catch a ball, or chase a pet around. The following interviews accent the love of movement, or play, which secures an athlete's long-lived physical activity.

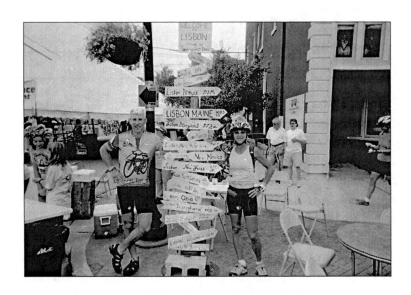

Robbi Young (on right).

"Well, why can't I?"

- Robbi Young

While I did not interview Robbi Young in person, I got to meet her at a launch party for my first book. Her vibrant energy was palpable. Robbi is a 51-year-old triathlete and marathon runner who lives in Erie, Colorado. When she was young, she participated in volleyball, basketball, and softball.

When in her mid-twenties, she discovered her love of running. In short order, she went from running 5K races, to 10K races, to half marathons, to marathons, and eventually to triathlons. Robbi has qualified for the 2010 Boston Marathon and is looking forward to finishing well there. Her impressive athletic history is possible because she always asked herself "Why can't I?"

She volunteers her time at events like the Wounded Soldier Ride and the MS150, a 150-mile bike ride fundraiser for the Multiple Sclerosis Society. Any excuses she has about succeeding in her sport evaporate when she sees the people who participate in those events. She says it is utterly inspiring to watch the wounded veterans who bike in the Wounded Soldier Ride persevere. And many riders in the MS150 are not highly trained. They just work hard to do the ride because they know someone with multiple sclerosis.

Q: You certainly show the ability to envision and then tackle a number of different sports. Explain how you got to be such a successful possibility thinker.

A: One day when I was debating whether or not to do something, a friend looked at me and said, "Why can't you do this?" I've carried that advice with me. When a friend calls and asks if I'd like to do a marathon, my thoughts are "Well, why *can't* I do it? What physical limitations do I have that makes it so I can't do it? What is in my way?" Unless I have a valid reason why I can't do something, I'll do it.

Q: You told me that you like to help people. What did you mean by that?

A: As I said, I do a lot of volunteer work for different events, but I also like to inspire and encourage people. I know how working out makes me feel; so good and healthy. I want to help others feel that way.

Q: What are the keys to your success?

A: I get a lot of good advice from coaches and other athletes. I did a one-hour lesson with a very good swimming coach, and he gave me excellent advice on the level of my hands in the pool. This little advice made a tremendous difference in my swimming. I also belong to the Boulder Striders running club, and we are coached by very qualified people who have taught me a more relaxed way to run. I also work hard. When I run, I run like I'm competing and I bike like I'm competing. I don't do leisurely rides and I don't do leisurely runs.

Q: What is your biggest challenge?

A: Time management. My mom has Alzheimer's, so between work, spending time with her, and training, time is pretty scarce. I plan my whole week in advance and use my calendar to schedule everything. I print it out and tape it on my desk so I know what I have to do and when.

"Just do your best and have fun."
- Bob Meluskey

Bob Meluskey Sr. is a 57-year-old dis-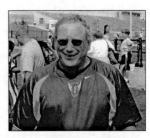
cus, shot put, and javelin thrower from
Wilkes-Barre, Pennsylvania. Bob has
participated in various sports his whole
life including baseball, slow pitch and
fast pitch softball, football, basketball,
track and field, motorsports racing,
hunting, and fishing. Bob very much values his family, which includes Sandi, his wife of 37 years, his son Bob Jr., and his grand-
daughter and fishing partner Samantha. He started competing
in masters track and field at the age of 51, when his wife kid-
ded him that he was over the hill. Far from it. In 2007, Bob was
nationally ranked 36th, 15th, and 11th in his age group for the
discus, hammer throw, and javelin events respectively. Bob is
an industrial maintenance mechanic who loves to work with his
hands, challenge his mind, and enjoy the camaraderie of masters athletics.

**Q: What do you currently do in your training that are keys to
your success?**
A: I do intense workouts keyed to my lifestyle and work ethic.
I like to workout. When it stops being fun, it's time to give it
up. I usually train before I start my work shift, which seems
to help with the stress involved in a high-end manufacturing
business where production is the only goal. It's hard being
on call 24/7.

Q: How do you set your goals?
A: When I compete, it's not for the medals or ribbons. It's about
the personal satisfaction that I've tried and done my best,
hopefully a personal best. If I medal, that's the icing on the
cake.

Q: What do you believe differentiates you from your contemporaries who aren't active?

A: I don't like sitting on my butt watching the boob tube, and my work ethic has me constantly moving, not sitting behind a desk. I use my hands and mind.

Q: Do you have a saying or motto that you live your life by?

A: "Just do your best." If I can look at the guy in the mirror and say I did my best, mission accomplished.

Q: Anything else you'd like to share?

A: To all masters athletes, remember this, you have to have a little bit of that kid left in you. Without that, it's no longer fun.

***

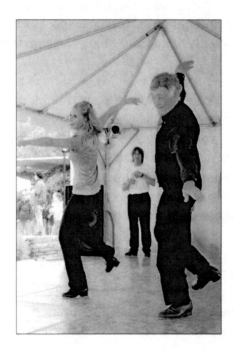

Gene GeBauer (on right) tapping with style.

"If the journey from Kamakura to Kyoto takes 14 days and you quit on the 13th day, you will never see the moon rise over the Kyoto."

- Gene GeBauer

This past summer, I was sitting around a campfire with some of my climbing friends discussing the athletes I was interviewing, when someone asked me whether dancers were athletes. I had never really thought about it, but as we talked about what it takes to be a skilled dancer and the physical nature of it, I decided that I would interview one. I'm glad I did.

Gene GeBauer is a 75-year-old tap dancer who lives in Denver, Colorado, and danced professionally on Broadway in New York City for many years. Growing up in Oregon, Gene played basketball in junior high school, but quit the team when he discovered dancing. He's forever grateful to Mr. Dimmit, the basketball coach, for supporting him in that decision.

Gene discovered dancing at 13 years old when his doctor suggested to Gene's mother that it could help him recover from rheumatic fever. He remembers enjoying the feeling of moving in patterns to rhythm, as well as the excitement of getting to dance with the girls. After his performing career ended, Gene became a dance instructor, and he still instructs today. Gene celebrated his 75th birthday recently, and former students came from as far away as New York City to celebrate the occasion and show him their appreciation.

Q: What is your biggest accomplishment in dancing?
A: It would be being successful on Broadway. Yes, I was a dumb kid who went from Oregon to New York City where I had no friends, but I wanted to dance and became a success. I'm also proud and somewhat amazed, that I maintained that success over 25 years, and worked with the biggest names on Broadway. I am happy to say that I have worked with Rogers and Hammerstein as well as the great dancer and choreographer

Gower Champion. My dance credits include *Camelot, Hello Dolly, Once Upon a Mattress, Sugar, Oh Calcutta*, and a show called *No Strings.*

Q: Goals in sports and dancing are probably different. How do you set dancing goals?

A: When I was younger, my goals were to be in a particular show or in a certain ballet company. When I was older, I wasn't a performer anymore so my goals shifted. I had a family and knew I was going to have to earn a living for the rest of my life, so my goal became to be the best tap dance teacher in at least a four- or-five-state radius.

Q: How are you dancing these days?

A: Not too long ago, Jason Samuel Smith, one of the best tap dancers in the world, was holding a weekend workshop and I got a chance to do a tap jam with him. We spent the evening jamming and afterwards he said to a friend of mine, "That Gene, he's cool. He's a cool cat. He dances so smooth and clear." I was tremendously flattered and realized I must still be pretty good.

Q: What was the best advice you were ever given?

A: There was a time when I was in New York and I became deeply involved in the practice of Buddhism. This particular sect was divided into men's and women's divisions, and we occasionally gave ourselves tasks that were literally impossible. Sometimes it involved very difficult physical things. I remember going to an activity where we did push-ups and chanted "Never give up. Never give up. Never give up," all together. You get tired, but when you're chanting "never give up," you keep going. I took that as advice and I don't give up so easily.

Q: Do you have a saying or motto that you like?

A: "If the journey from Kamakura to Kyoto takes 14 days and you quit on the 13th day, you will never see the moon rise over the Kyoto." This has had a great influence on me. It means that if you set a goal and you quit before you attain it, you will never experience that which you said you wanted to experience.

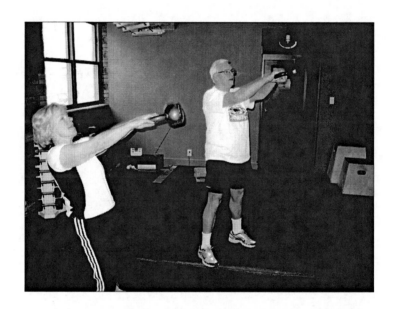

Louise and George Thornton staying strong together.

"Do now what others won't, so later you can do what others can't."
- George Thornton

"I love it because I feel good as I train. I physically feel good and I mentally and emotionally feel good."
- Louise Thornton

It can be challenging for a couple to dedicate themselves to active lives. Time and energy can become scarce and the demands of training can put strain on a relationship. Despite some of these issues, George and Louise Thornton have found that their life together is enhanced by the physical activity that they share. George is 69 and Louise 67, and they currently enjoy triathlons, including the grueling, full Ironman distance.

George is a retired college professor who participated in many sports in his childhood, but focused on swimming, his strongest event, until he went to graduate school. In grad school, he picked up handball and played regularly until his mid-forties when he saw a newspaper article about a masters swimming event. Feeling a bit burnt out on handball, he decided to rediscover swimming. A couple of years later he did his first triathlon and since then has completed more than 90 of them.

Louise, who has master's degrees in audiology and theater, played golf, tennis, and softball in her youth. As an adult, for fitness reasons she began running with a friend. She discovered that she really enjoyed running and went on to compete in masters track and field sprint events. Having always loved golf, she tried to get George to take it up, but to no avail. She decided that if she and George were to spend more time together, she had to take up triathlons, and she did.

Q: **What has playing sports together meant to you?**

Louise: We have a really good time traveling together, going to various races, and meeting new people. We socialize with a great set of new active athletic friends. We also encourage each other and feed off each other's energy in training.

George: We don't normally train together very much, but last year I was returning from a shoulder injury and Louise had signed up for the Canada Ironman. We trained together quite a bit then and it was great. Years ago we did multi-day bike rides together, such as Ride the Rockies and Pedal the Peaks in Colorado, as well as rides in France and Italy. We really enjoyed those.

Q: **You mentioned a three-day event where you both did five endurance races. What more can you tell me about that?**

George: Maxomania was the name of it, and it was held for two years in central Missouri. The event was for couples and we were the oldest married couple.

Louise: It was for pairs of all sorts. Two men, two women, married couples, etc., and they were in different categories.

George: It started with a triathlon on Friday afternoon, followed on Saturday with a triathlon, a duathlon, and swim or run. The grand finale was an Olympic distance triathlon on Sunday morning.

Louise: St. Charles, Missouri is where it was held – in the woods. Nearly everyone stayed at the resort and ate dinners together there. It was a great time.

Q: **You both look fantastic and are in terrific shape. What sustains you?**

Louise: I think it is the cross-training. It is the fact that we run, swim, bike, and do other things. This helps us stay fresh and avoid injuries for the most part. I also just enjoy training. It makes me feel great.

George: I also really enjoy working out. I have goals and like to compete, but that alone wouldn't sustain me. I also like it when I tell someone that I just did a triathlon and they are amazed that I can still do that at my age. I like the notoriety, but that certainly wouldn't sustain me either. I think it boils down to enjoying workouts.

"I absolutely love the sport. I love the motion of it. I love its simplicity. I love the freedom of running."
- Susan Henderson

Susan Henderson had a very modest start as an athlete, but kept working at it, and went on to enjoy quite a bit of success as a runner. She is now surrounded by fit, healthy people in her job at Adidas, a company best known for their athletic shoes.

Susan, 62, lives in Lake Oswego, Oregon, and got her start with running in 1969 when she saw an advertisement for Dr. Kenneth Cooper's book *Aerobics*, on the back of a margarine package. I'm sure she never suspected that margarine would play a role in turning her into a lifelong runner. Dr. Cooper's program clicked with her immediately, and she began taking her young son to a nearby track where she could keep an eye on him while she ran. Before she knew it, she had improved and was running a mile in 6:30.

She later saw an advertisement for a marathon and decided to try it, despite not knowing that a marathon was 26.2 miles. Nonetheless, she completed that race and was hooked. Eventually, she qualified for the first women's Olympic Marathon Trials in 1984.

In addition to running, Susan also enjoys cycling, hiking, and lifting weights. Having had eight years away from racing, she has set some new goals and is looking forward to getting back into it.

Q: You've been running for a long time. What keeps you motivated?

A: First, I'm lucky that I've stayed healthy and have never had any major injuries. Second, I absolutely love the sport. I love the motion of it. I love its simplicity. I love the freedom of running. I love getting on a trail and running for a long time. I like that running allows me to be competitive. With the person in front of me that I'm trying to catch, the person behind me that I'm trying to hold off, and with myself when I'm out there trying to get a personal best time on my favorite route.

Q: What have you done to remain injury free?

A: I really listen to my body. I do whatever it takes to be able to keep running and often that means letting my body recover. I make sure that I take at least two days off each week. I know I'll never run as fast as I used to and I'm good with that, as long as I can continue to run and stay healthy.

Q: What do you still hope to achieve?

A: My ultimate achievement would be to remain healthy for the rest of my life and be able to continue doing the things that I enjoy. One thing athletics does is make you think about the way you eat and how you treat your body. I'm so happy that I found running as a young woman and that I have been able to continue doing something that I love so much.

Q: Where do you draw your inspiration from?

A: I've always gotten my inspiration from my late father. He and I were really close. He had been a professional boxer and was a scratch-handicap golfer for many years. I caddied for him while growing up and I saw what it took to win; he was very competitive. I grew up with his attitude for competition. He taught me to work really hard and not back down, and he's the person I would think of when I stood on the starting line of a race.

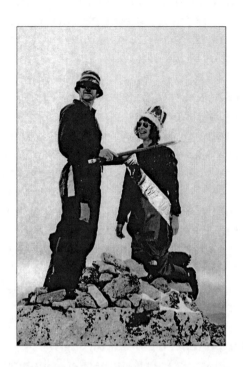

*Jean Aschenbrenner, Queen of the Colorado 13ers
(photo by David Kennison).*

"Just get up and do it!"
- Jean Aschenbrenner

Jean Aschenbrenner is a 61-year-old rock climber who lives in Boulder, Colorado, and was the first woman to climb all 637 of Colorado's mountains over 13,000 feet in elevation. While in high school, Jean visited Colorado as a prerequisite so that she could travel to Europe with her Girl Scout troop.

It was on that trip that Jean reached the top of her first 14,000-foot mountain, Pikes Peak, and fell in love with the mountains. She did rock climbing for the first time when she was in college, and recalls how she loved the feel of the rock and the physical challenge. After college, Jean spent time in Kenya with the

Peace Corps and climbed many peaks during her time abroad. Following her work there, she came back to Colorado where the mountains have, once again, captured her imagination and given her countless days of joy.

Q: Climbing 637 peaks in Colorado over 13,000 feet is incredible. What motivated you?

A: Part of it is setting goals and making it happen. Besides that, I love doing it; I love the challenge – that's probably it. Physical challenge is always what's given me the most joy in life.

Q: What sort of training do you do for rock climbing?

A: In the winter, I climb pretty regularly in the rock gym because I love going there. I like the feel of climbing as well as the social aspect. I used to run to keep in shape, but now because running is hard on my joints, I go for very fast walks. It's a great workout.

Q: Have you experienced a breakthrough?

A: I was once in Joshua Tree National Park climbing with a friend of mine, Mark Nelson, who is a much stronger climber than I am. After Mark reached the first ledge where we paused, he told me that he wasn't sure he could do the second pitch, because the first pitch really tired him out. In that situation, either I had to lead the next pitch or we needed to rappel to the ground.

Because I didn't want to go down, I decided to try and lead the second pitch, which traversed around a corner and was quite intimidating. I had never led anything that hard. So, I led partway out, and then I came back to the ledge, completely controlled. I rested a bit, then led back out, and up around the corner to the next ledge. I did it! After that, I had way more confidence in leading harder stuff. It was Mark's belief that I could lead that pitch that led to this breakthrough.

"It's not training, it's play!"
- Rich Davis

Rich Davis is a 54-year-old triathlete who lives in Fort Collins, Colorado, and has been doing triathlons from the very early days of the sport. Rich swam competitively from a young age up through college, and after college took up cycling and running.

One day in 1979, after he had done a 5K swimathon and afterwards rode his bike 50 miles to his sister's house, his sister showed him a *Sports Illustrated* article about the first Ironman triathlon. He figured that he had almost done one that day, and decided to compete in a triathlon. Rich went on to have lots of success in triathlons and marathons, and even won a Canadian National Ironman Championship triathlon.

He says he does not train for events, but instead considers his workouts play. Ken Kelly, a swim coach, got him started swimming at age eight. Rich gives Ken tons of credit for introducing him to a life that he loves. He recently called Ken and told him how much influence he had had on his life.

When Rich told me this in our interview, I decided to follow his example, and called my high school cross-country coach Dave Doak. I thanked Dave for teaching me how to dream, set goals, work hard, and celebrate. I'm glad I called when I did, because Dave and his wife were preparing to relocate, and I may have not been able to find them. I think that everyone who has had a coach or someone who helped get them started should call to thank them today. Don't wait. They deserve more thanks than we can ever give them.

Q: What do you currently do in training that is the key to your success?

A: It's never training for me, it's playing. I think of what I do as play. I'm just goofin' around with a bunch of buddies, doing cool things and checking out interesting places.

Q: How do you set your goals?

A: I've never really looked for goals; they've presented themselves. For example, I got back into swimming after a three-year break, and my goal became to survive the college swim season. Another time I decided to avoid a dead-end career and go back to school. At first, I planned to take a few courses in computer management, but after the first semester my goal became to get the degree.

Q: You've been active for so long; how do you do it?

A: For me, being active is a lifestyle. I can't imagine not being active, maybe because I've been active since I was eight years old.

Q: What was the best advice you were ever given?

A: In life, anticipate where the next great place is going to be, so you can be there first. I did that with my work in computers as well as in doing triathlons. Being able to see the next big thing puts you ahead of the pack, whether it's in sports or in a career.

Q: Where do you draw your inspiration from?

A: I draw inspiration by watching special Olympians compete. That is the purest form of sportsmanship.

***

As we can tell from the interviews, these athletes have a deep love for their sport or activity. We can see it in the way they view exercise as fun, the way they persevere in their sports, and the way they play at their exercise. Their instinct to play is perhaps the most important ingredient in their sustained active life.

If openness to having fun and engaging in play is so important, how do we improve our ability to add more to our lives? Try the *Do It!* exercises on the following page for ideas and suggestions.

[1] Medic, N., Starkes, J. L., Young, B. W., Weir, P. L., and Giajnorio, A. 2005. Master athletes' motivation to train and compete: First order themes. *International Society of Sports Psychology (ISSP)*, 11th World Congress of Sports Psychology, Sydney, Australia, 1, 1-3.

Do It! Exercises
Love It

- Make time for physical play. It's more important than you may think; how can you put a value on joy and a strong, healthy life?

---

o How much time each week or month do you devote to this kind of play?

---

o How much time are you willing to set aside for active play?

Make it a priority by scheduling time for it each week or month. Schedule this time the way you would any other activity. You owe it to yourself to have a good time!

- Need ideas for playful activity?
  - o Chase your dog around. (Chase a cat and you'll really get a workout!)
  - o Play with your children or with kids in your neighborhood. They are ALWAYS willing! Do whatever game they come up with.
  - o If it's snowing, build a snowman or igloo. Make snow angels, or go sledding.
  - o Make a play date. Ask your friends if they want to come and workout with you. Everyone wants to play. They are probably waiting for an invitation.
  - o Try something new with a friend. Sign up for a dance lesson, do Zumba (aerobics with Latin music), yoga, or take your dog to an agility contest.
  - o Look in your local newspaper for events or ask around. There are lots of active things going on, and you just need to make a little effort to find them.

- Question your self-image.

  - o List the exercise activities that you associate with your self-image.

o List the activities that you would like to do that are not consistent with your current self-image.

o Pick one of the above activities and ask yourself what it would be like if you did it anyway.

If the implications of doing this activity are acceptable to you, arrange the opportunity and *Do It!*

- Reconnect with play that you once loved doing.

o What types of exercise and play did you enjoy when you were a kid?

o What activities can you do at your current age and in your current situation that have some of the characteristics of the activities you liked when you were a kid?

Pick one of the above activities and try it for a few weeks.

Over-50 athletes are primed for play. Play through movement. What a good excuse to goof around. What great fun to laugh with friends while building strength. With play as an incentive, who could resist loving their workouts? Not so fast. There's one more thing to consider: solidly integrating physical activity into our lives.

Chapter 5: Live It

"Continuous effort – not strength or intelligence – is the key to unlocking our potential."
-Winston Churchill

We've seen that it is critical to envision ourselves as living an active life and to discover a physical activity that we love to do. It is equally important to follow-through and incorporate being active into our daily lives, to *Live It*. Having completed the Performance-to-Transition lifestyle, the 50 athletes have this step under control.

To find out how they do this and what techniques they use, I posed several questions in the surveys. I examined their answers to see how they *Live It*, and distilled their collective wisdom into summaries and statistics that can help us understand this process. The first question was:

1. *What things are you currently doing in your training that are key to your success?*

The highest number, 34 percent, of the 50-plus-year-old athletes said the most common key to success in training was consistency. Even though I was under 50 at the time, I can relate to this. When I was running competitively in high school and college, I used to take off large blocks of time. I would sometimes take the entire summer or winter off, with the thought that I would return rejuvenated and ready to work hard again. Doing this seemed to work well when I was younger.

Now that I am 46, I see the wisdom of exercising consistently and not taking big blocks of time off as we get older. The past few years, I took November and December off from climbing, and I found that whereas this let some of my little aches and pains heal and subside, it was very hard to claw my way back into shape.

With a score of 10 percent, "recovery and listening to my body" was the second most important key to success. This makes sense to me, as I believe that the frustration associated with injury keeps many people from participating in sports when they get older. Several of the athletes told me that when they were younger, they would workout very hard and not require much recovery time. At that time, if they did become injured they would heal much more quickly than they do now.

The need for more recovery time and the need to listen to our bodies circles back to the need for consistency. If injured, they won't be able to exercise regularly. This is good information, even for those of us who have not yet reached 50. It reminds me of that wonderful visual of the tortoise and the hare: the cautious and consistent tortoise is able to achieve what the impatient hare could not.

Older athletes acknowledge their limitations, but they don't limit themselves too much. They may not be as *fast* or *strong* as they once were, but that doesn't mean they can't go as *far* as they once did. It's a different pace, and that is all right for Performance-to-Lifestyle Transition athletes, because this is what it takes to continue living a strong, healthy life.

2. *What differentiates you from contemporaries who have tailed off in athletic participation?*

Love for being active and love for their sport was the response. Having already analyzed why athletes in this group love their exercise, this is no surprise. Younger athletes may feel an obligation to physical activity, may act out of hero worship, may workout primarily to look good, or have some other external motivation. Over-50 athletes are in it for the love of doing it.

That love is in line with what they indicated was the most important joy; the joy of movement. We recall that loving a sport, starts with the ability to listen to the childlike urges for seeing possibilities and for engaging in play. This playful state of mind then leads to movement, and it is movement that yields to love of the sport or exercise. When we engage in this process, we are happy captives to one of the best things that could happen to us later in life.

3. *How do you set your goals?*

The most common response to this question was given by 24 percent of the athletes. They said that they don't seek challenges as much as they let challenges come to them. They said that if the opportunity presents itself and it sounds like fun or sounds interesting, then they may take it.

What this tells us is that they are generally no longer so intensely competitive, that they want to set performance-based goals. They have a relaxed, playful approach that is in line with the importance of maintaining a balanced and active life. This approach results in their taking on new challenges and experiences that just look like good fun.

Another way that over-50 athletes said they like to set sports goals is to arrange training around a calendar of annual events that they like. Many tailor their yearly training around a few key events, using other events in between for preparation and conditioning.

4. *What is your biggest challenge and how do you manage it?*

Finding the time to train and compete, received 26 percent of the vote, and so did staying healthy and injury free. Predictably, respondents who were not yet retired, have job and family responsibilities that can crowd out their recreational time. Those who struggle with the sense that time to exercise is scarce said that in order to manage, they try to find balance and try to have clear priorities. They often "pencil in" workouts on their calendars just as they do other commitments.

Those who felt that staying healthy and injury free is their biggest challenge said that they are cautious about fitness and pay attention to their bodies' needs. They also take care of themselves by regularly visiting doctors for check-ups.

5. *What is your diet like and how did you come to integrate it into your lifestyle?*

When asked to describe their diet, many said that they were not on any special diet. It is true that the diets they describe are quite varied and are not bound to a certain regimen, but what's striking is how healthy the diets are compared to the average American diet. Most avoid junk food and fast foods. Many avoid red meat. Many take some sort of supplement, such as vitamins, glucosamine, or protein shakes. Most all have a diet rich in vegetables and fruit. Again, that's because these athletes have found an activity that they love to do and realize they need to have a strong, healthy body to be able to do it. A good diet seems to go with the territory, since they automatically take great care of themselves. Their interest in eating well is almost intuitive.

Mental Tips for *Living It*

A good number of the over-50 athletes said that they depend on visualization, or *Dreaming It*, for their athletic success. Terry Peterson told me that this is critical for him to be able to do the outlandish jumps that he performs on a unicycle. He sees himself accomplishing what, to others, looks impossible.

To add to our *Dream It* conversation, visualization can take many forms. Maybe we simply glimpse ourselves performing a new activity, or have an idea that a different sport would be fun. Such thoughts can be fleeting, however. Repetition is known to bring the best results. There is a difference between briefly thinking that it would be fun to ride a bobsled, and the demanding visualization drills used by Olympic bobsledders.

Along the spectrum between a fleeting fantasy and an intense mental drill is an effective visualization technique for reaching your goals. I call it Writing It Down (WID). Many, many athletes have used this technique to their advantage. There is something very powerful about having to refine a goal to the level of specificity required to write it down, and then actually putting it on paper. Recording a goal makes it more definite and helps to bring it into reality.

As an example, I was on a college cross-country team, when my teammates and I convinced ourselves that we could place in the top five in the NCAA Championships. The only problem was that we had never placed higher than 18th. That summer, I made up posters that said "Top 5 in '85" inside an outline of the map of the U.S., and mailed them to each person on the team. Everyone proudly displayed the posters in their apartments. That year we went undefeated in the regular season, and finished 3rd in the championships. If you employ no other visualization technique, I suggest you use WID.

The concept of never giving up, also surfaced many times in the interviews. I have not counted the number of times the phrase "never give up" was uttered to me, but it probably is right up there with "I love it." With so much at stake for older athletes, they know that giving up their tenacity in even the small things could mean a slippery slide on a downward slope. It's extremely important to them that they steady their resolve, hold to their goals, and consistently workout. Never would they want to have a weak body. Never would they want to be more prone to illness. Never would they want to give up their satisfying, active life.

With so much at stake, the mental and physical tips they shared with us are important and have proven to work for the majority of the athletes. We can follow their lead by using this advice, which includes scheduling regular workout times, paying attention to any strain that we put on our bodies, and doing exercise for the love of it, rather than for other reasons. These next interviews will give additional insights into how some of the athletes *Live It*!

***

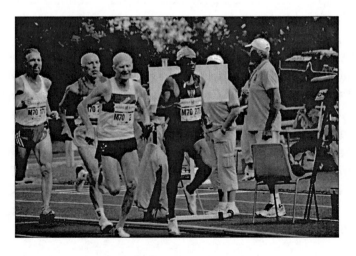

Sid Howard (far right runner) in the lead.

*"If you don't hold your head up so high in victory,
you won't have to hold your head down
so low in defeat."*

- Sid Howard

His warmth and desire to help anyone and everyone makes Sid Howard well-known among masters track and field athletes. At 70, he runs track, cross-country, and road races from his home base in Plainfield, New Jersey. Excelling in high school track and cross-country, Sid was a talented runner from the start. He told me that he also excelled at being the class clown, which in the 11th grade, led to low grades and being bumped off the team.

When he was 39, a friend told him about a masters race that was being held at a nearby school and he rediscovered running. Sid was surprised that they had races for people who were out of school, and signed up. He's been racing for over 30 years now and recently won the gold medal for the 1500-meter event at the World Senior Games in Lahti, Finland.

Throughout all of the interviews that I conducted, only a few things amazed me. One was that Sid said he does 500 sit-ups each day. And he's 70 years old! That blows me away. Go Sid!

Q: You took a long break from running, so when did you realize you could be a champion?

A: After eight years of running competitively. I was 47 years old. I was running in the national championship two-mile race and won the gold medal. In that same meet, I won the mile and half-mile races, so I went home with three gold medals. It wasn't like "I gotta win, I gotta win," it just happened. That day changed my life. I realized that I am a champion and now approach every race that way.

Q: So, how do you set your goals now?

A: I try to set goals based upon what I feel, but if I set a goal and I don't achieve it, it's okay. It used to drive me crazy if something came up that made me miss a workout. Now, if I have to miss a workout, I figure it is what God meant to be, and I'm okay with it.

Q: Any tips for younger runners who would like to stay with it for a long time?

A: I used to run a lot of miles on the concrete and asphalt, but have switched to running mostly on dirt, grass and the track because it is easier on my joints. My 500 sit-ups a day have given me core strength that I need in the later stages of a race when my arms get tired. I started by doing 25 sit-ups per day, and when I worked up to doing 100, I couldn't believe it. Now I do two sets of 250. I also do a significant amount of running sideways and backwards to help stabilize my muscles.

Q: What was the best advice you were ever given, and who gave it to you?

A: My grandfather told me, "If you don't hold your head up so high in victory, you won't have to hold your head down so low in defeat." That has helped me through every failure I've ever had. You always have to give good grace to your competitors because without them, there would be no race.

Q: What do you tell people who want to be more active?

A: I'd like them to realize that they don't need to be a runner or cyclist to become more active. All they have to do is to get moving. Get moving, not for other people, but for yourself. It doesn't mean that you will live longer, but as long as you do live, you'll be healthy.

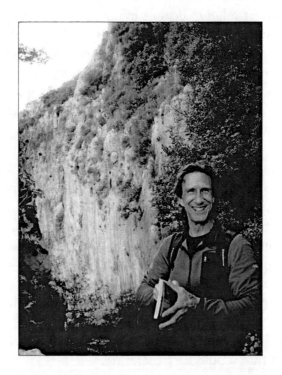

Russ Clune at the Crag (photo by Amy Pickering).

**"It's always later than you think. When you die
and you have work left on the table and money in
the bank, you've run out of the most precious
thing: time. Don't waste time doing
stuff you don't want to do."**

- Russ Clune

When I used to live and climb in New York, I would occasionally see Russ Clune climbing in the Shawangunk Mountains. Russ was older than me and a much better climber, and he would often climb with those who were younger than me. I never dreamed that someday I would interview him for a book.

Russ is a 50-year-old rock climber, who lives in New Paltz, New York. He has traveled to dozens of countries to climb, either for pleasure, or for his job as a sales representative for the climbing equipment manufacturer Black Diamond. Russ remembers participating in swimming and golf at a very early age, and became interested in the adventure of camping and hiking when he was eleven. He was enamored with the classic alpine literature of the time, and loved the wild feel of high places.

In the first week that he attended the University of Vermont, he had the chance to rock climb. Once he did, he knew he had found his sport. In time, he traveled the world and climbed leading-edge routes, always enjoying the people he met along the way. The only other sport he has ever done that engaged him like climbing, is surfing, which he picked up when he lived in California. Back in New York now, Russ works at finding balance among his job, his family, his friends, and climbing.

Q: I recall seeing you climb with younger climbers. It seems to me that that would be frustrating.

A: I embrace the younger generation and set my ego aside. The young climbers are incredibly motivating for me. I try to suck power out of them. I have friends who continue to climb, but they do the same routes they've done many times. That's okay, but I like to keep pushing myself, and I get great motivation from the younger climbers.

Q: You've traveled extensively for climbing. What was that like?

A: Back in the early 1980s, I spent six years climbing full-time and got to travel all over the world. I met a great variety of people, and got to do world-class level climbing. I got to watch sport climbing explode around the world and that was incredible. I think that experience is my biggest accomplishment.

Q: **Are there any climbs that stand out in your mind as break-throughs?**

A: In 1983 I did a route named Vandals with Hugh Herr, Lynn Hill, and Jeff Gruenburg, and it was the first route with a rating of 5.13 in the Eastern United States. That was a break-through, because it was the hardest thing in the east at the time, and also because it was a team effort by the best climbers in the area. Who did it first was not the end all. We all must motivate each other to do our best.

In 1994, shortly after I moved back to New York from California, I got reenergized by climbing. I was working another difficult climb called Mantronic with my friend Jordan Mills, and I felt really far away from doing the crux move. Jordan would tell me how close I was, and made me believe I could do the route. He pushed me, and supported me, and I eventually did it.

Q: **What things do you believe differentiates you from your contemporaries who have tailed off in their athletic participation and abilities?**

A: For many of my buddies, climbing was a means to an end. Climbing helped them lose weight or get some sort of gratification, and then they moved on. For me, climbing has always been a lifestyle.

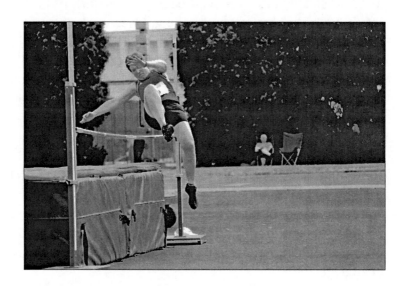

Kim Williams clearing it!

> *"The will to win is nothing without the will to prepare."*
>
> **- Kim Williams**

Kim Williams is a 54-year-old sprinter and jumper from Portland, Maine. When growing up, her school didn't offer much in the way of sports opportunities for girls. Inspired when she was 35 years old by a group at work who ran at lunchtime every day, she hopped on the treadmill and ran for 20 minutes. She remembers telling one of the runners that she did this, and the woman told her she was off to a great start. That small bit of encouragement changed Kim's life. She started running and went on to do road races until 2006 when she discovered the sprints and jumping events in track and field.

A fellow runner told Kim she would be a great addition to their company's corporate track team, so she started running their mile and two-mile races. She entered some shorter races to gain points for the team, and discovered that she was quite talented. She broke the team record for the 100-meter run in her fourth 100-meter race. Since then, Kim has taken up high jumping, hurdling, and even experimented with the javelin throw. With her love of learning and trying new things, she hopes someday to compete in a pentathlon.

Q: Who are your role models and what motivates you to do your sports?

A: I've got great role models. I know athletes who are very accomplished and talented in all age groups. When I first got into masters track and field, I expected that the 90-year-old athletes would just be out there doing it for fun, but they're out there running, jumping, and throwing their hearts out. It occurred to me that the body ages, but the competitive spirit doesn't.

People may think that we're just doing our sport as a lark, but we're just as serious as any other athletes. We're just in older bodies. I recall that right before I turned 50, one of my aunts asked me if I was nervous about being that old. I told her that she should meet the 50-year old women that I know. They're beautiful, talented and athletic. Two of my friends climbed Mt. Kilimanjaro last year, so they're not women that are sitting around knitting. Not that I have anything against knitting.

Q: You mentioned that you love to try new things. Can you give an example?

A: I never thought I could high jump because people told me it would be hard to get over the fear of jumping with your back turned. But I told my coach that I wanted to try it for a meet, so he gave me a few lessons. At the meet I made the low height, the next height, the next height, and beat a woman that I considered to be a good high jumper. I found that I really liked high jumping, and now it's one of my favorite events.

Q: What was the best advice you were ever given?

A: A marathon runner from Kenya who won the Boston Marathon a number of times said, "The will to win is nothing without the will to prepare." I think that I've always remembered that, because you can want to win all you want, but it's the getting out there day after day and training that makes it possible.

Q: Do you have a saying or motto that you live your life by?

A: I often think of that George Sheehan's saying about every runner being an experiment of one.

Q: Where do you draw your inspiration from?

A: My inspiration is definitely from my competitors and the older women. We compete fiercely against each other, but it's a very supportive environment.

Q: Anything else you'd like to share?

A: I'm hoping that your book about athletes over-50 will give a good look at what many older athletes are doing. Occasionally, I see an article about an older athlete, along the lines of *Those Amazing Animals*, which almost holds them up as some kind of weirdo. I just wish that people realized that 11,000 people went to the National Senior Games in 2007. I was ripping mad one day after I read an article about a guy who was overweight and planning to do a marathon. That same week a friend of mine broke an age group world record, and it didn't even make the paper. Why does someone who's planning to do something get more publicity than someone who's actually doing it? That's the end of my little rant.

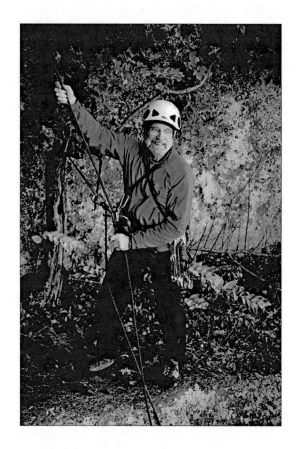

George Hurley enjoying belay duty (photo by Anne Skidmore).

*"I'm inspired by the fun of climbing, the fun of
adventure, the fun of exploring, and by
finding something new to climb."*

- George Hurley

George Hurley is a soft-spoken, 74-year-old rock climber and ice climber who lives in Wonalancet, New Hampshire. George has established hundreds of new rock and ice climbing routes across the country since the 1960s. In high school he ran track and played football. He began climbing when a graduate school classmate took him climbing up Cussin' Crack in Boulder Canyon, Colorado. He liked it so much, that he became a climber that day.

George taught English at the high school and college levels, and in 1974 switched from teaching English to teaching and guiding rock and ice climbers. He was a guide in Colorado for several years before moving to New Hampshire where he has been guiding for various organizations ever since.

George also establishes new climbing routes in New England, and he loves the adventure of seeing a new line and finding out whether he can climb it or not. I plan to take him up on his offer to climb with him the next time I am in New England. Being a climber myself, I appreciate George and others like him who spend countless hours finding, cleaning, and making new climbs available for others to enjoy. Thanks George!

Q: There is a saying that "there are no old, bold climbers," but seriously, how have you kept at it for so many years?
A: Over time, many of my contemporary climbing friends have found other interests. In my case, I'm still very enthusiastic about rock climbing and ice climbing. Managing to stay healthy has helped me stay with it. Another factor is that I haven't had children. Many climbers with children do continue to climb, but others find that family and job take all their time and energy. Since 1974 my profession has been

my sport.

Q: What about your climbing are you most proud?

A: My biggest accomplishment is the many new routes that I have established. I've been regularly putting up new lines since the 1960s. I haven't kept count, but they number in the hundreds. In the old days, when I was establishing new routes in Colorado and Utah, it wasn't as difficult as it is to-day.

Today, especially here in New England, it's a lot of work. I'm working on a new route right now and it's covered in lichen with dirt in the cracks. I've had to rappel with a wire brush and clean it. It used to be easy. It used to be that you could walk along a cliff like Lumpy Ridge and do things like the George's Tree climb from the ground up. You'd just start at the ground, go to the top, and you'd have done a first ascent.

Q: Have you experienced climbing breakthroughs?

A: I've had many breakthroughs; mostly connected with im-provements in equipment. For instance, when I started climbing, we'd tie the rope once around our waists. Well, somebody said, "Hey, if we have to hang on the rope, it would be a lot more comfortable if we could put this around two times?" Then came the harness, what a wonderful break-through! In ice climbing, I started climbing with a straight pick, and the ice axe was mainly a cutting tool; you cut steps in the ice, and climbed. You couldn't climb vertical ice with a straight pick. When the reverse curve ice axe came along, we could easily climb things that were impossible before. I was in my late forties when sticky rubber was first put on climb-ing shoes. What a difference that has made.

Q: How do you train for climbing?

A: I don't really do much training. I've been doing yoga for more than 25 years, and my wife and I practice at home twice a week. We also like ballroom dancing. If there's no dancing to be done out and about, we dance in the kitchen. I was at an American Alpine Club party last Saturday night, and there was lots of dancing. It turns out that there are not many men who like to dance, so I get lots of exercise! I'd been climbing all day, and then I danced until late in the evening. I think it's really good fun, and good training.

Q: What inspires you?

A: I'm inspired by the fun of climbing, the fun of adventure, and the fun of exploring. I like the people I climb with, and I like being a guide because I learn new things from younger guides and from my clients.

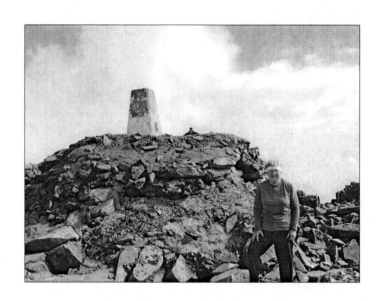

Barb Page hiking the Scottish Highlands.

"Retirement means more time to train."
- Barb Page

Barb Page is a 71-year-old runner and Nordic skier who lives in Fairbanks, Alaska. She taught high school chemistry, and when asked by her students what she would do when she retired at 67, she told them she was going to get back in shape and do a marathon again. I imagine that those kids were pretty well astounded when she said that.

When Barb grew up in the 1950s, there were not many opportunities for women in sports. She played basketball in high school, and was even made captain of the team her senior year. In college, she played on the girl's varsity basketball team, but did not get a varsity letter because at the time, female athletes were not eligible for varsity letters. But in 2007, Barb's college alma mater presented Barb and her teammates with their varsity letters to celebrate the 25th anniversary of Title IX legislation, and that is a memory that Barb will always cherish.

While teaching in Alaska, Barb was introduced to Nordic skiing by a fellow teacher, and she has skied ever since. In 1966, a friend asked her to hike the Fairbanks Equinox Marathon, and Barb finished in 11th place. She figured that if she could place 11th by walking, maybe she could do really well if she ran, so she ran the same marathon a year later. From that point on, Barb continued to run and ski. When she retired in 2005, her training really kicked into gear. Her log shows that she skied 377 miles in the winter of 2005/2006, 428 miles in 2006/2007, 515 miles in 2007/2008, and 345 miles in 2009.

Q: What do you currently do in your training that are keys to your success?
A: Just getting out there and doing it! I just love the feeling of being out there. It's just great! I don't need to enter any ski races, because the skiing is very fulfilling on its own. I also don't over train. When my body tells me it has had enough, I listen

to it.

Q: What would be your ultimate achievement?
A: I would like to still be running, skiing, and hiking when I'm 90. I'd also like to hike the Chilkoot Trail, which is the trail that people who followed the Klondike gold rush took from Skagway, Alaska, up over the mountains into the Yukon Territories. It's an amazing, steep, and difficult 33-mile trail.

Q: How do you set your goals?
A: I'll see something in the paper or hear about something and decide to try it because it sounds challenging and fun. In 2007, I went to Scotland for a family gathering with my brother and his wife, and I found out that Scotland's highest peaks are called Munros, which is one of my ancestral names. Then we decided to climb Ben Nevis, the highest mountain in the United Kingdom. Climbing that mountain was the hardest thing I have ever done. It was harder than a marathon because it was very steep and had rough terrain.

Q: What is your biggest challenge?
A: Staying injury free. This summer, forest fire smoke is also a big challenge. I've got a 16-mile race coming up and we've been having such heavy smokes that there are warnings not to go out and exert yourself.

Q: What was the best advice you were ever given?
A: Get some decent running shoes! I did my first marathon in hiking shoes, and the only other option I had was high-top basketball shoes. One of my students was a runner, and he said, "Mrs. Page, you've just got to get some good running shoes!" And I did. My first shoes were Bangkok Roadrunners, and I ordered them from Blue Ribbon Sports in Eugene, Oregon, because I couldn't get them in Fairbanks. My son also told me to get some modern base-layer clothing for skiing, and some modern ski boots. Man, what a difference that made. I can ski when it's 15 and 20 below now. Oh, it's just wonderful!

Q: Anything else you'd like to share?
A: I consider myself a mediocre walker and runner, and there are lots of people who are better. I just like to do it, and I've discovered that I have practically no aches and pains, my weight is under control, and my mobility and balance are very good. I *like* it!

***

The interviews we just read, are from people who have given us clues about how we can deeply integrate sports or exercise into our lives. Maybe some of their techniques will be useful to you. Below, you can answer the same questions that they did, and mull over whether or not some of their clues might give you an advantage.

Have some fun with the following Do It! Excersies on the next page!

Do It! Exercises
Live It

- What things do you currently do in your training that are key to your success?

- How could you be even more successful with your training?

- What differentiates you from your contemporaries who have tailed off on athletic participation?

- How do you set your goals?

    o If you're not already doing so, would you like to let your goals "come to you?"

- What is your biggest challenge and how do you manage it?

- What is your diet like?

  o How could you improve your diet?

We can learn from the 50 athletes who integrate these tips into their lives, because they know how to keep a successful athletic program going after the age of 50. They tell us that consistency in exercising and staying injury free underscore success, while goal setting tends to be more relaxed and based on enjoyment. The biggest challenge to routine exercise for those over-50 is staying injury free. Incorporating visualization, especially through writing down our goals and having a "never give up" mindset, are beneficial in living a life of athletic success when we're older.

Our over-age-50 athletes have given us all of these suggestions and so much more to work with. Having followed the sequence of *Dreaming It, Loving It,* and *Living It* towards a strong and healthy life, what is there left to do? For some people, it's *Giving It.*

Chapter 6: Give It

"Your most precious, valued possessions and your greatest powers are invisible and intangible. No one can take them. You, and you alone, can give them. You will receive abundance for your giving."
-W. Clement Stone

This chapter is devoted to the generous athletes who took the opportunity to give back and help others live better lives. To be sure, there is a lot to be gained from volunteering. In giving back they were able to share their talents, meet interesting people, see new worlds, and, of course, feel good about their contributions. But in the end, these over-50 year old athletes looked around and found that they could use their skills and caring hearts to help others in need.

If they followed the pattern of volunteering in the U.S., they would have donated an average of about one hour a week, and would be very glad they did. A study conducted at Washington University in St. Louis, Missouri, polled 401 volunteers over 55 years old.[1] It showed that 30 percent claimed they were "a great deal better off" due to the services that they donated.

Interestingly, where health is concerned, a few hours spent volunteering can also be an ounce of prevention. What really took me aback was the disclosure in this study that *20 percent had "improved overall health"* as a result of volunteering to help others. It looks like those who couple a little volunteer work with their exercise plans, might have even more of an edge on good health.

Healthy Reform vs. Health Care Reform

After I had completed 20 of the interviews, I experienced an un-expected detour in my journey. My wife Sylvia was volunteering; she had offered her restaurant as a drop-off point for a food drive. I went out for a run and my mind drifted to how one of the oldest athletes I interviewed said he is not on a single pre-scription drug. I was again reminded about how all the people I had interviewed seemed in extraordinarily good health.

Then it hit me. Suppose I could somehow combine the volun-teer work I'd like to do with my book project? Suppose I could do something about "Healthy Reform," rather than health care reform? I'd long thought that America wouldn't have as large a health care crisis if, through exercise, we could each take re-sponsibility for reforming our health.

50-K Active/Athlete Challenge is Born

That is when I had the idea to recruit 50,000 people to adopt some of the healthy habits I had documented from the inter-views. I named this effort the 50-K Active/Athlete Challenge. Our mission is to recruit 50,000 people to adopt these five sim-ple, healthy habits by 10/10/2010:

1. Move! Find a sport or physical activity that you LOVE to do
2. Set a goal and write it down
3. Make a plan to reach the goal and write it down

4. Set up a way to be accountable
5. Get out there, follow your plan, be accountable, and have FUN!

Folks can register on www.50-k.net, the 50-K Active/Athlete Challenge website. By registering, you are not only taking a step to improve your own health, but also making a statement about the importance of an active life through Healthy Reform. The site provides members with inspiring and educational articles; the chance to interact in forums; get support from each other; and be rewarded through contests and in other ways. With more Healthy Reform, America will need less health care reform!

The interviews that follow may stir you to follow suit, and start giving back in some way. If so, the *Do It!* exercise at the end of this chapter may prove helpful.

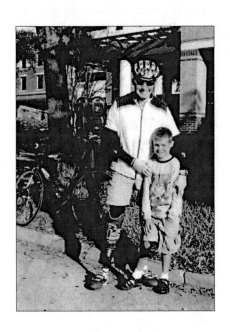

Bill Hansbury (left) with his friend Jake.

Bill Hansbury:
Helping amputees regain an active life.

"Boston Bill" Hansbury's story is a testament to the power of being receptive to opportunities. A 72-year-old cyclist and runner, Bill lives in St. Petersburg, Florida. He became active at the age of 28 when a friend he hadn't seen in awhile visited. Bill asked his friend how he managed to look so great, and his friend replied that he had taken up running.

Bill jumped up, went to his bedroom, put on some sneakers and said to his friend, "Let's go!" Since that time, he has been running regularly, stopped smoking, and lost a lot of weight. He got so good that he ran an under-three hour marathon. He also performed in ultra-marathons and took up cycling.

Unfortunately, a couple of years ago Bill lost a leg to an aggressive, antibiotic-resistant infection. Recently, he has been helping others with disabilities to live a better life by helping them get prosthetic limbs.

Q: Your story is remarkable and touching. How did you come out from an amputation, feeling so strong?

A: After my amputation, I remember sitting on the edge of the hospital bed, looking down, and seeing that my foot was gone. In the hospital, I did a lot of thinking about what I was going to do, and I vowed that I would get back to running and cycling as quickly as possible. I wasted little time with regret or sadness over losing my leg.

I decided that I would use the technology that is out there and treat that prosthetic leg just like it's my real leg. The day that I came out of surgery, I called a friend that was a wheel chair athlete, and asked him if he would please have a hand-powered cycle waiting for me when I get out of the hospital. He did, and after I got out, I was on it within a few days. Since then, I've been able to resume regular cycling as well as running.

To help amputees obtain prosthetic limbs, I created the Boston Bill Foundation. It is an interesting story how I came to this. I had finally gotten back to where I could ride my bike comfortably, and headed out one morning for a group ride. I've used clip-in pedals for years, but at one point on that ride, I could not get one of my shoes to release from the pedal. A couple guys who were on the ride grabbed me to keep me from falling over, while they worked to free my cycling shoe and my foot. They ended up taking my foot out of the shoe because it was stuck in the pedal.

It was quite an ordeal, and when the shoe finally came free, I sent the other riders on while I regrouped. That's when a man and woman pulled up in a car and said, "We saw you with your prosthetic leg on the bicycle and we wondered if you would talk to our son Jake. He is seven years old and we are on our way to the children's hospital. He is going to have his leg amputated this morning."

Jake had been run over by a riding lawn mower three years before, and his leg had sustained major damage. He had undergone a series of operations, but he still couldn't play with his friends anymore. His parents had been struggling with their decision to have his leg amputated, and seeing me that morning, a 72-year-old man with a prosthetic leg – riding a bike, they felt they had made the right choice. I agreed to speak with Jake, and when we were done talking, they went on to the hospital and the little boy had his leg removed.

Somehow, the *St. Petersburg Times* picked up the story and did an article about Jake and me. Later, *People Magazine* did a photo shoot of us. One day I got a call to come to San Diego and present a prosthetic running leg to Jake. To see him run and play now is extremely touching for me.

One other thing is that, you can believe what you want, but that shoe had never stuck in my pedal before or after that day. For some reason, on that day, at that time, it got caught, and brought Jake and me together. I created the Boston Bill Foundation to help others with disabilities live a good life through exercise.

Q: Since losing your leg, what about running has changed for you?

A: When I was in the hospital, they spoke to me about phantom limb sensation, and kept telling me that it would eventually go away because your brain doesn't realize your leg is gone. That seemed so silly to me. I thought that if I had a leg for 70 years that it would be crazy for me to want that sensation to go away. So, I started doing little exercises, like tapping my heels on the floor, both of them at the same time, and letting the sensations travel up my leg. There's a series of six exercises that I worked out for myself and I still use them every day.

As a result of these exercises, when I ride a bicycle now, my right leg and my left leg feel exactly the same. I can feel the pedal and I can feel the pressure in both feet. I try to teach this to some of the other amputees that I deal with. When they do these exercises, it also gives them a sense of feel that helps them walk better, climb stairs better, descend stairs better, ride a bike or even run.

Q: What is your biggest challenge, and what do you do to manage this challenge?

A: My biggest challenge is in doing very long rides or runs, as I am still learning about my prosthetic. I need to make sure the equipment I'm wearing is up to the task. It would be a bad situation to be out there, break a piece of equipment and not be able to replace it. I'm learning how to deal with this on a daily basis.

Q: Where do you draw your inspiration from?

A: My inspiration comes from inside me. When I was 11 years old, I remember getting ready to deliver newspapers early one Sunday morning. It was raining and snowing at the same time, and I had a load of papers in a sled that was so heavy I could barely move it. My dad had just come home from a long days work, and I remember going in to ask him if he would come out and help me.

He told me, "You go out and do your job; I just finished mine." I was so mad, that I went outside and I moved that sled, and was able to complete the paper route that Sunday morning. Every time I go to do something difficult, I think of that day; I go and I pull the sled. I thank my father every time I remember that day, because he did me a big service by enabling me to be strong.

***

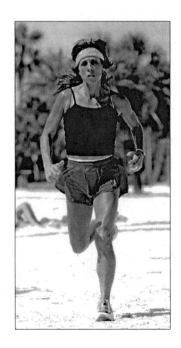

Myrna Haag running strong.

Myrna Haag:
Helping people break food addiction.

Myrna Haag and I spent the first 30 minutes of our interview calming ourselves down because we were both so enthusiastic about helping people to lead healthier lives. Myrna is a 50-year-old triathlete who lives in Tampa, Florida. She was on the swim team in high school and took up running in her late twenties.

It was then that she discovered triathlons, because someone in her town told her about races in which you ran, cycled, and swam. Myrna did a local sprint triathlon and won. Her second triathlon was a half Ironman and to her surprise, she qualified for the Kona Ironman in Hawaii. She eventually ranked fourth nationally.

Despite this success, when I asked her about her greatest accomplishment, Myna told me about her mission to help others. For more than 20 years, she has helped overweight people by teaching them how to view food differently and how to become active.

Q: Tell me about the breakthrough you had with that?
A: I was in my mid-thirties when I discovered that I had a real purpose, which was using my gift for motivating people to eat well and be active. At one point, I became aware that I had this gift, and realized that with it I could help many people. I've always loved teaching people and getting them to be active. People were giving me great feedback about this and some even told me that I totally changed their lives.

Q: What is your biggest accomplishment?
A: I've done athletics for years and have been pretty successful, but I feel that my greatest accomplishment is helping people to improve the quality of their lives.

For a long time, it's been my mission to help those who are overweight and don't have the means to learn how to be healthier. I'm talking about people who can be 100 pounds overweight and who can't move like you and I do. It's almost like they are trapped in their own flesh, and I teach them how to get their bodies in balance through improved nutrition and movement. I've probably worked with several thousand people in the last 20 years. I've written a book about the program I have developed for them. It's titled *Six Steps to Never Diet Again: Free Yourself from the Diet Trap*.

Q: How do you sustain your motivation?

A: I absolutely love working out and feeling my muscles work. I don't know for sure, but I have this feeling that many people who have stopped, never really loved it. I think that some of them did sports for reasons other than the pure joy of it. It may have been something on their to-do list. I've known women and men who were great athletes, then stopped and gained 50- to 60-pounds.

Q: What do you currently do in your training that is key to your success?

A: I try to work my muscles every single day. I will go out and bike, run, swim, or do calisthenics for at least two hours a day. I work muscles all over my body. I just love the all-over feeling of my muscles working, even more so if I am outside. I just love being outside in the elements, feeling that feel.

Q: What was the best advice you were ever given?

A: "The real secret of success is enthusiasm." Enthusiasm is bigger than intelligence and it's bigger than wealth. Nothing great has ever been achieved without tremendous enthusiasm. I'm sure Albert Einstein didn't say to himself "today I sort of feel like working on that relativity thing." No, you have to be crazy mad! You have to be over the top. You almost have to be obnoxious.

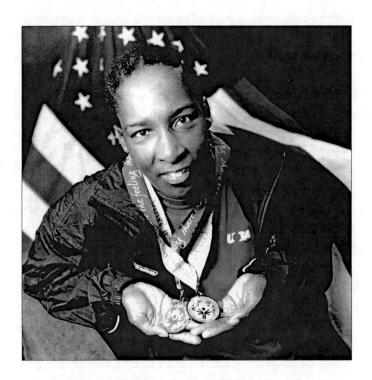

Loretta Caliborne, Special Olympic Champion
(photo by Schintz Studios of York, Pennsylvania).

Loretta Claiborne:
Ambassador, Special Olympics.

Loretta Claiborne is a 56-year-old runner and inspires people through her work with Special Olympics. She lives in York, Pennsylvania, and when she was 12 years old her older brother introduced her to running. Since then, Loretta also participated in ice skating, bowling, tennis, snow skiing, basketball, and golf.

One day, she discovered the Special Olympics when someone in a workshop at her high school noticed her running rather than taking the bus to school. That encounter opened up a world for Loretta that led to a lifelong love of sports. She would eventually run 26 marathons, one of which was the Boston Marathon. Running has become a part of her daily life, and she even uses it for transportation around town. Now she is trying to become a better tennis player.

Q: In sports, what is your biggest accomplishment?

A: Some people might think that running the Boston Marathon or going to the Special Olympics World Games might be my biggest accomplishments, but I think it is that I am able to run like I do, despite several surgeries on my feet and legs. Some people told me I would never run again after the surgeries, yet here I am today, still running. I love that I am making my dream a reality. I love being the athlete that I want to be and being a Special Olympic athlete.

Q: What sport is your current focus?

A: Aside from the running component of my training, I lift weights and do stomach crunches at the community center. I run about an hour a day. It's part of my transportation. Recently I needed to go get a flu shot, so I ran to the clinic and got one. Some people hop in their cars, but I hop on my feet!

Q: How do you set your goals?

A: I believe that if I train hard enough, if I focus, I can prevail. A few years ago I decided that I wanted to play tennis. In 2008, I went to the Special Olympics State Games with the goal of winning one tennis game. I took the skills test and did well, so they matched me against the top girl in the state. My goal was to win one game and I ended up winning two. My goal this year is to be competitive with this girl and win the first four games. My goal next year might be to beat this girl. It's not the medals. It's about beating this young lady to prove to myself that I have the ability to do it.

Q: Do you have a saying or motto that you live your life by?

A: So much emphasis these days is put on winning and on the elite athletes. We can just be ourselves, and that's enough.

I use the Special Olympics motto "If I can win, let me win; if I cannot win, let me be brave in the attempt." I also use the motto "God is my strength and Special Olympics are my joy." In Special Olympics, not only do I have the opportunity to do a sport, but I get to meet people, and we laugh and have fun.

Q: Where do you draw your inspiration from?

A: I draw my inspiration from the likes of Eunice Kennedy-Shriver, who created Special Olympics. She gave many people, who would never otherwise have had the opportunity, the chance to experience the joys of sports. I met her once. She came up to me, put her arm around me, and said, "I want to be like you." I turned to her and said, "If only I could be an eighth of what you are, and what you do for humanity."

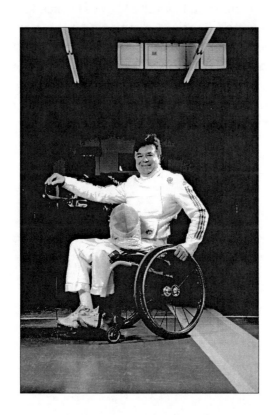

Gerard Moreno ready to bout.

Gerard Moreno:
Helping paraplegics adjust to their new lives.

Gerard Moreno is a 52-year-old Paralympian who lives in Los Angeles, California, where he operates his own accounting business. Gerard has a quiet confidence around him, and his quiet tone is amplified by his powerful words. While growing up he played football, track and field, snow skiing, and fencing.

At the age of 18, he suffered a gunshot injury, which left him partially paralyzed. After about six months, Gerard ventured out and tried playing wheelchair basketball with a team at the hospital he went to. He loved seeing that he could enjoy sports again despite his injury. Amazingly, he went on to take up water skiing, tennis, downhill off-road wheelchair racing, and scuba diving.

Doing these sports enhanced Gerard's self-confidence, and has led to a life full of fun and adventure. These days, his focus is on basketball, off-road racing, and fencing. He has been on the United States Paralympic fencing team three times and won numerous national championships.

My interview with him was very inspiring because he not only has an extremely positive attitude, but he is also on a special personal mission. He gives back to recently-injured athletes who are making the transition to new lives. He learns how to adapt to new situations. He passes this lesson on by volunteering.

Q: You're very accomplished in a number of Paralympic sports. What are your sports and exactly what have you accomplished in them?
A: In downhill wheelchair racing I was national champion for three years. In fencing, I've been national champion seven times. In wheelchair basketball, we went to the final four in 2001 in the Paralympics.

I'd say the best competition I had was in the Sydney Olympics. It was probably the best moment in my life as far as accomplishments go. It was my first Paralympics, and I was the last person to fence on the saber team. We had a fence-off with the team from Kuwait, and the winner advanced to the final eight, while the loser went home. I was last of the three people on my team to fence, and we were down terribly, 33 to 40. In these matches the first team to get 45 points wins. For some reason our coach chose me as the closer, which is unusual because typically a coach would choose an "A" fencer, a person who has significant abdominal mobility and is usually one of the strongest fencers.

We were in one of the larger pavilions in Sydney, and the place was packed with avid fans. When the match started, my opponent and I scored four touches on each other fairly quick. It was 37 to 44. Somehow, at that point I got in "the zone" and started making one touch after another. I was just whipping this guy. I scored the next 8 touches on him and we beat the Kuwait team 45 to 44. The place erupted. It was just incredible.

Q: What is your biggest challenge?
A: I have a problem of not staying in the present moment and sometimes letting other outside factors get into my head while I am in competitions. So my biggest challenge is being present and not letting the umpire or my opponent shake me. I read a book titled *The Power of Now* by Eckhart Tolle; it was extremely helpful in getting me to remain in the present.

I discovered that it's important to be concise, clear, and focused on your objective, and to not let anything else get inside your head. It's about not thinking. You can't be thinking about your dog, your wife, your mom, your work – nothing. During competition, I think to myself, "This is what I am going to do. I'm here and I'm in the moment, and I'm just waiting to unleash what I am here for." When I can do this successfully, my opponents have no chance of defeating me. I'm just going to go through them like a blow torch through butter. But it's very counterintuitive and very difficult to master.

Q: How have you managed to stay active for so long – especially being partially paralyzed?

A: I think it's my attitude. I have never lost that kid-like mentality for competition, having a good time, and playing. I feel it's a great benefit to be able to stay in great health by playing a game. I think that keeping your child-like person in the forefront of what you are doing is really, really important. I do have more responsibilities now. I am older and have a house, a wife, and all of the responsibilities that go along with being at my stage in life, but I still feel like a kid.

I also have learned to adapt. Being active yet physically hurt, I had to adapt to a whole new lifestyle. I believe that the person that can adapt most easily and continue to fight is a person that's going to prevail.

Q: Do you have a saying or motto that you like?

A: "It's the journey, not the destination," because I have had so many incredible experiences on this journey as a Paralympian. I've been to incredible places and met great people. I've been able to mentor and set an example for a lot of people. For example, I've done sports clinics for newly injured vets, and it meant a lot to me to help them find a new sport and a new way to get back into life.

Q: Anything else you'd like to share?

A: I just wish everyone was as fortunate as I am. A lot of people look at me in my wheelchair and can't understand my positive attitude and outlook, but I've got to say that had I not been hurt, I probably wouldn't have the same philosophy of life. I feel very blessed to be part of a national team and the Paralympics' team. Plus, I find joy in other people and in being on this earth.

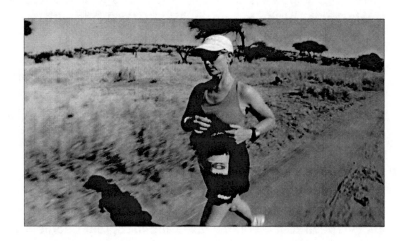

Linda Quirk running "down under".

Linda Quirk:
Helping people with addiction recovery.

Linda Quirk is a 56-year-old marathon runner who splits her time between her homes in California and Jacksonville, Florida. A retired school teacher, Linda has been active her whole life, but had not participated in competitions until age 35 when her brother asked her if she wanted to do a marathon with him. Not a 5K or a 10K, but a full marathon. They ran their first marathon together that year, and Linda was sold. She ran a number of marathons after that, and eventually took up Ironman triathlons.

A bad cycling accident in 2005 had Linda returning to marathons as her primary activity, and boy has she! Linda runs marathons all over the world, in part, because she has made fundraising for the Caron Foundation her life's purpose. The Caron Foundation is the fundraising arm of a group of drug and alcohol rehabilitation centers.

Q: Tell me about how you got started doing events for charity?
A: In 2005, I was on a 100-mile bike ride and had a catastrophic accident. I fractured just about every bone in my head. I was in the intensive care unit for three days and I'm lucky to be here today. After the accident, everyone was telling me to give up triathlons. My heart was telling me that I needed to get back on the horse and ride. I had already qualified for the world championships in Sweden that year, and I wanted to be there. So I went, without the blessing of the neurologist, and did well.

I then felt that I needed to qualify for the Kona Ironman Triathlon, and I told myself that if I did, the only reason I would race from then on would be to give back. I have a stepdaughter who was addicted to methamphetamines, and we had lost her to the streets for three years. We had just gotten her back and she was in recovery. I wanted to do what I could to help others who are struggling like she had. We are here for a reason; I really honestly believe this is mine.

To qualify for Kona, I did a triathlon in Lanzarote, Spain, which is more difficult than Kona. The winner of that race qualifies for Kona, and I came in second. Lucky for me, the woman in front of me declined the invitation to Kona, so I got to go. I was able to raise $50,000 for a scholarship fund for people who can't afford drug and alcohol treatment. My focus now is getting people to look beyond themselves and give back by doing something good.

Q: Traversing four deserts is a mindboggling feat. How did you come up with that fundraising idea?

A: I like to reach beyond, and tried to do that even when I taught school. The kids would usually reach the goals I set for them, or ones they set for themselves. My motto is "Dream Big." I truly live by that. I did the Kona Ironman and thought, what could be tougher than that? Then I saw that people ran seven marathons on seven continents, and thought that sounded cool. So I did it, raising $294,000 to help even more people who cannot afford the addiction treatment they need. Then I thought, well, I've never done an ultra-marathon, so I'm doing my first one in October. Next year I'll tackle four deserts. I love dreaming big.

Q: Can you tell me a little more about the desert adventure you have planned?

A: I'll be attempting to run the four deserts in a year. I would be the first women to do this, unless another woman sneaks ahead of me. If someone does, at least I'd probably be able to say I'm the oldest woman to do it. I'll do the Atacama Desert in Chile, the Gobi in China, the Sahara in Egypt, and finally the desert of Antarctica.

Q: What was the best advice you were ever given?

A: My first triathlon coach told me that the minute you put your foot in the water, you've finished. You won't turn back. You're going forward and not thinking about it anymore. To this day, the minute I take that first step, I know I'm going to finish.

Q: Do you have a saying or motto that you live your life by?
A: If you can see it, you can do it; if you believe it, it will happen. So dream big.

Q: Where do you draw your inspiration from?
A: I draw a lot of inspiration from my husband. He's absolutely been my rock and someone who came from nothing to create a wonderful world for himself and his family. He's always laughing and always happy. He can see the humor in everything. He's my biggest inspiration.

* * *

The people whose interviews you just read have taken the step to give something back, because they feel very fortunate to be living strong, healthy lives, and because they want to share their good fortune with others. So now you know a little about some good causes that you could support! Or, if you are moved to give back and need some help figuring out how, complete the following exercises.

---

[1] Morrow-Hollow, N., PhD. February, 2009. *The Gerontologist*. Vol. 49, No.1: 91-102.

Do It! Exercises
Give It

- If there is a cause or problem in your community that you are passionate about, what is it?

- What tools, skills, or resources do you have that you think would be useful in helping this cause (knowledge, training, personal or professional network, computer skills, money, time, property, etc.)?

- What would it feel like for you to apply the resources that you have to help your cause?

- If giving back is still something that seems rewarding for you, list actions that you can take in the next week to find opportunities to get started.

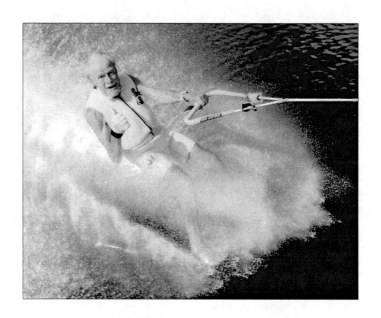
*Banana George shows how it's done at
age 91 (photo by Lynn Novakofski).*

Chapter 7:
The Ultimate
Over-50 Athlete:
"Banana" George Blair

"If I have seen further than others, it is by standing upon the shoulders of giants."

-Isaac Newton

There is no one who exemplifies a strong and healthy life better than 94-year-old "Banana" George Blair. World-renowned for his colorful athletic style, George discovered a passion for water skiing in his forties, and developed an exercise plan that has served him into his nineties. He was still water skiing, barefoot, at the age of 93.

It was my good fortune to connect with George and his wife JoAnne. I am honored that George gave me his approval to include this profile of him in my book, because he is the very definition of what an older athlete is capable of.

If Jack LaLanne is the pioneer of raising America's awareness of what can be achieved through fitness, it is Banana George who symbolizes the joy and exuberance available through exercise. All who know the love of an active life owe a tremendous amount of thanks to both George and Jack for helping to stoke the fire of our athletic passions.

George's life is as interesting as it is long and strong. Born in 1915, he grew up in Toledo, Ohio, and was captain of his high school golf team. At Miami University of Ohio, he studied government and political science. With the Great Depression in full swing, George would hop trains to get from Ohio to Florida for spring break with his college fraternity brothers. It was on one of these trips that George was thrown from a train by hoboes and badly injured his back. This unfortunate incident would actually set the stage for the invention of Banana George as we know him.

After college, George worked for the city of Butler, Pennsylvania; served as a procurement officer in the Army Air Corps during World War II; and started a company that took hospital photos of newborn babies and their mothers. Later, as a successful banker and real estate investor, he lived in New Jersey and had an apartment in New York City. In his late thirties, his back injury was so painful that he needed to have surgery. After surgery, he spent time recuperating in Florida.

His doctor advised him to swim to help him recover, but when George tried, he sank like a rock. A water ski instructor suggested that he try skiing, and when he did, George became totally enamored with the sport. At age 46, he skied barefoot for the first time, and soon adopted the moniker "Banana George," because of his lifelong love for the color yellow, his love for bananas, and the sunshiny joy that he himself exuded when he water skied. From yellow wetsuits to yellow suit jackets, George can readily be seen wearing his trademark color.

With his newfound enthusiasm for skiing and his knack for showmanship, George was soon entertaining crowds at Cypress

Gardens in Florida. He was so adept at water skiing that he set several world records, including being the oldest person to ever barefoot water ski. He was also the first person to barefoot water ski on all seven continents.

Known all over the world, George has been a guest of leaders of many countries, including China, Australia, France, Germany, and Monaco. His popularity proved itself with American women when in 2002, *Sports Illustrated for Women* voted then 87-year-old George one of the world's sexiest men in sports!

Having picked up one of his fondest sports at the age of 46, George represents an approach to exercise that is taken by the majority of the over-50 athletes I have interviewed. This approach is used by innovative people who change from one sport to another – sometimes more than once. The result is a fresh and interesting physically active life.

George often tried new athletic adventures. After skiing barefoot for the first time at 46, he took his first solo airplane flight at 53. Then at 70, he took up wakeboarding; at 75, snowboarding; at 81, race car driving; at 82, skydiving; at 83, surfing; and at age 85, he rode a bull.

It's been said before: he's an incurable daredevil. Couple that with his outrageous joy and enthusiasm, and it's easy to understand his legendary influence on American athletics. George's vitality has infused our culture with a "can do" spirit for decades, while his playfulness reminds us of the fun and pleasure that we get from sports. Who in America's athletic community hasn't been affected by his crazy-happy spirit?

George, we thank you from the bottom of our healthy hearts!

Chapter 8:
The Experts Weigh In

"I look upon every day to be lost, in which I do not make a new acquaitance."

-Samuel Johnson

In process of developing this book, I was fortunate to connect with Dr. Nikola Medic, Ph.D., and Dr. Vonda Wright, M.D., two well-known experts who have devoted many years of their lives to studying different aspects of aging athletes. Their in-depth psychological and physiological research, and their insights on athletes and aging are presented in the following two chapters.

I happened upon Dr. Medic's work while I was researching the sports motivations of older athletes. Dr. Medic is a lecturer in sport and exercise psychology at Edith Cowan University in Perth, Western Australia. He has published 12 book chapters and journal articles and has given more than 40 presentations at professional and academic conferences throughout the United States, Canada, Australia, Asia, and Europe. His research focuses on a variety of issues related to sport and exercise psychology, which include motivation, talent development and identification, mental training for elite sport performance, and well-being. Over the past eight years, he has served as a sport psychologist consultant to individual athletes as well as to various teams. He has also presented numerous group workshops.

In the following chapter *Dream It, Live It, Love It: the Research Evidence*, written by Dr. Medic himself, he shares psychological and behavioral research that coincides with the key messages in this book. His contribution is a substantial enhancement to this work and will be of interest to those who want to delve deeper into the research literature that he offers.

Dr. Vonda Wright, is an orthopedic surgeon, speaker, and author, who conducts medical and physiological research on masters athletes. One of the few women in orthopedic surgery in the United States, she specializes in sports medicine and is the director of the Performance and Research Initiative for Masters Athletes at the University of Pittsburgh Medical Center. In these roles she cares for athletes and active fitness participants over 40; from people stepping away from the couch for the first time in 20 years to weekend warriors and elite competitors. She also conducts research on athletes over 40, as well as on musculoskeletal aging. As an expert in maximizing performance and minimizing injury in adults, Dr. Wright penned her first book, *Fitness After 40: How to Stay Strong at Any Age*, in 2009.

Dr. Wright, who authored my later chapter entitled, *How Fast Do We Age?*, shares with us some of what she has found in her own research, as well as what other studies have shown regarding the ability of the human body to perform athletically as we age. Her summary is both enlightening and inspiring.

Chapter 9:
Dream It,
Live It, Love It:
the Research Evidence

by Dr. Nikola Medic, Ph.D.

The interviews conducted with 50 athletes over 50 contain major themes, which for the most part, are supported by the empirical literature. The key messages conveyed in this book are, in my opinion, of crucial importance to any middle- to older-aged individual who is interested in improving his or her physical health and well-being.

There are also certain psychological motivators and sociological behaviors that are known to encourage continued healthy athletic activity. A closer look at these gives us a greater awareness about how we can commit to successfully continue our athletic involvement, and can help us understand what might strengthen our continued participation in sports. The psychology and sociology information that I review enhances the major themes that emerged from the investigation into the lives of the over-50 athletes.

Insights and data from my past and current research on masters athletes, as well as from sports psychology labs worldwide, provide a psychological and sociological context for the research conducted for this book. The insights that I present come from a variety of sources, including my sports consulting experience, and my research based on archived records of more than 40,000 masters athletes in addition to my survey data on more than 600 masters athletes. The athletes possessed different ability levels in bowling, golf, marathon running, athletics, and swimming.

Training Consistently While Staying Injury Free is Crucial

Throughout the book, consistent training for older athletes was identified as vital to gaining the most long-term exercise benefits. Being consistent requires moderation, life balance – and most importantly – staying injury free. To find how this is done, I examine the rates of age-related decline in physical performance and review evidence on how such decline can be tempered through continued physical training. I then evaluate evidence on how much training may be helpful to gain optimum benefit, and what kind of training a typical masters athlete does. Understanding factors that moderate age-related declines is important to effectively and efficiently assist aging individuals with their training. Even more important, from a psychological perspective, is how understanding these factors can help us accept that decline in athletic skills is inevitable as we age.

Can Exercise Affect the Natural Aging Process?
The deteriorative effects of aging are demonstrated in a wealth of research literature. Patterns of age-related decline have been well documented for memory, aerobic capacity, maximal heart rate, muscular strength, and flexibility, to name a few. Although physical aging effects are irrefutable, there is some question as to how much these pronounced trends reflect primary aging, and how much inactivity or "disuse" exacerbates these trends.

Many theorists have argued that athletic trends for age-related decline are pronounced due to declining involvement in a sport or to insufficient athletic practice. Thus, one avenue of research has been to examine age-related patterns of training and performance from populations of highly active and sufficiently practiced individuals such as masters athletes.

Various approaches, like analysis of cross-sectional, longitudinal, and world-record athletic performance data, have been taken so that we may understand the effects of continuous lifespan sports on the aging processes of masters athletes. First, researchers empirically describe their observations of age-related rates of decline in performance for masters athletes, and then contrast these rates with figures believed to represent normal aging trends. Generally, these studies suggest that after the peak performance age of 35, performance gradually declines at .5 percent to one percent per year until approximately age 70 when the decline accelerates. Some studies also suggest that the rate of decline differs as a function of event, sport, and gender. For example, the rate of decline is generally greater for distance than for sprint events, for swimming and athletics than for golf, and for women rather than for men. Another avenue of research concentrates on comparing various characteristics of masters athletes to population norms and to inactive individuals.

By and large, these studies indicate that many age-related changes have been found to be less pronounced in masters athletes. As a result, the lack of physical activity in older adults is becoming widely accepted as a primary contributor to decreases in functional capacity and increases in morbidity and mortality.

What Type of Training is Important and How Much is Enough?
Whereas chronological aging is inevitable, to a certain degree training is under the control of the individual. This assumes that they are motivated; have access to equipment, coach-

ing, and facilities; are able to remain free of injury; and are not compromised by the effects of "secondary processes" of aging. An example of a secondary aging effect might include the self-damage that arises from prolonged training over many years that may hinder the opportunity to train later in life.

To examine the degree to which the typical decline in 10K running performance of middle-aged masters athletes age 40- to 59-years can be slowed, my colleagues and I collected longitudinal performance and training data from 30 runners. Our results showed that those who retained the highest level of performance, or had the smallest declines in performance over a period of 20 years, were succesful because they maintained years of uninterrupted practice, consistently had shorter off-season periods, exhibited higher weekly amounts of sport-specific practice, and *avoided injury*.

Other research found that masters athletes are more likely to experience acute and chronic injury, to have a fear of injury, and take longer to rehabilitate than younger athletes. Further support for the importance of staying injury free comes from one of my research studies conducted with more than 300 masters athletes from swimming along with track and field. Here I found that the most commonly reported reason for having lapses in motivation to train occurred after an injury. Comments from participants included, "An injury breaks my routine," and, "It happens on occasions when I am exhausted, worn out, super tired and still trying to run when I really need an extra day of rest." This study also showed that even though the majority of masters athletes have no intention to quit training and competing in the near future, most said that injury would be the most likely cause for them to stop.

In terms of the amount of training and the number of competitions that masters athletes do, studies have found that they generally spend quite a bit less time practicing than younger elite athletes. Masters athletes actually average about seven hours per week, which is on average approximately 50 percent less practice time than younger elite athletes. However, it is interesting that the structure of their practice, which includes warm up, flexibility, speed, endurance, technique, and weight training, is very similar to that used by the younger elite athletes. My research also revealed that masters athletes attend an average of five competitions per year.

Schedule Training Around One or Two Major Competitions

One unique finding from the research conducted in this book is that masters athletes structure their training around one or two major annual competitions that they consider to be of upmost importance. This finding is interesting for at least two reasons. First, research shows that masters athletes consider their "performances" at competitions, such as their running times, as more successful than their "outcomes", such as their ability to place at events. They also believe that their performances are a more direct result of their own internal resources and intentions than their ability to place.

In addition, my research tells us that masters athletes report high levels of task goal orientation and a moderate level of ego goal orientation. By definition, those with a high task goal orientation are more likely to see themselves as competent, because they tend to judge their performance in self-referenced terms and because they are prone to feel autonomous, since they get more satisfaction from mastering a sport skill than from attaining a certain standard of performance. On the other hand, masters athletes who are high in ego goal orientation tend to be more interested in anticipated outcomes such as rewards and acknowledgment, rather than the inherent aspects of sport or the mastery of a task. Together, these results suggest that focusing on performance to attain a certain time, for example, rather than focusing on outcomes like winning medals or defeating others, may give masters athletes more gratification and help them sustain their involvement in sport.

The second reason that masters athletes structure their training around one or two major competitions relates to my research findings on how masters athletes perform in their age group. Findings based on the analysis of archived data on more than 40,000 participation entries from 1996 to 2007 and more than 2,000 national records set from 1998 to 2007 at USA Masters championships in athletics and swimming, show that masters athletes are more likely to enter and perform well in competitions when they are in years one or two of a five-year age category.

Masters Athletes Are Highly Competitive

Another common theme in this book is the extremely competitive nature of masters athletes. Although helpful in mastering their sport, competition can be a challenge, since these athletes often have a hard time accepting age-related declines in their performance. To compensate, some switch to new events and/or sports, but there are at least two other successful strategies that can be used. Mentioned by numbers of athletes interviewed in this book, one strategy is to use goal setting as a tool to help reassess long-term goals. For many, being able to continue sports participation beyond their 70s or 80s is much more important, at least in terms of their health and well-being, than being able to maintain or improve performance and/or win medals.

The second strategy involves using age-grading tables that have mathematical formulae based on archival performance data, to get age-corrected times from absolute performance times. Age-grading tables are currently available for athletics and swimming. An advantage of the age-grading tables is that a performance level percentage (a higher percentage indicates better performance) can be calculated and used to compare performances across a wide range of events, independent of a person's age. Another advantage of using age-grading tables is that a person's current performance can be compared to previous performances regardless of age, because all are mathematically converted to age 35. For example, in absolute terms it may look like an athlete's current running time is slower than the time he achieved five years ago. However, the mathematically adjusted time with his age factor removed could show that his running performance has actually improved.

Intrinsic Motivation and the Importance of Enjoyment

Of primary importance in this book is the data showing that before they could get truly involved with an activity, the 50 athletes thought of the opportunity as an enjoyable experience. It was also noted that once an engaging activity is found, the ability to maintain enjoyment and develop commitment and passion for their sport creates the momentum required for constant training and involvement. To discover how these characteristics can be successfully integrated into athletic life, I reviewed the research literature, which I believe can assist aging individuals find effective and appropriate motivational strategies to support their continued, successful sports activity.

Research studies show sports participation and physical activity generally decrease with age. In North America for example, participation rates in competitive sports show a pattern of decline after individuals reach their twenties, and by the age of 50, only 1 in 10 are motivated to be involved in sporting activities at least once per week. Research also indicates that more than 50 percent of the people who start an exercise program drop out after only six weeks, suggesting how hard it is for many to maintain even a minimal exercise routine. Finally, considering the increasing number of seniors in the general population, understanding what motivates masters athletes can give us strategies that could be used to help our older population be more active and healthy through sport.

How Masters Athletes First Get Involved in their Main Sport

In one of my studies, my colleagues and I surveyed over 450 masters athletes from athletics and swimming. We found that there are three most common ways through which they enter into masters sports. These were through continued involvement in competitive sports, through their social network, or through community recreational activities. In this survey we found that 49 percent had been consistently involved in their sport since they were young, and 22 percent had switched from one sport to their current sport. Of those who used recommendations from their social network as a means to begin a sport, 18 percent received recommendations from a doctor, 15 percent from friends, 10 percent from family members, and 8 percent from a coach.

Lastly, of those who started a masters sport through masters athletes' community recreational activities, 9 percent started as the result of being a fan, coach, or official; 21 percent started after becoming a member of the community sport programs or a local masters club; and 9 percent began when they learned of opportunities through the local media.

What Motivates Masters Athletes to Continue to Participate in Sports?
A number of studies conducted to date, including the research reported in this book, show that regardless of sport, masters athletes have a variety of motives for continuing to participate in sports. These include enjoyment of the sport, opportunity to test skills, health and fitness reasons, social reasons, and extrinsic rewards. In addition, several studies have shown that self-determined motives, which are a part of a person's innate character, can also be a primary motivation for continuing to train and compete. To this point, there is evidence that most masters athletes are very self determined, goal oriented, and do not intend to stop participating in sports.

There are also other studies that suggest that masters athletes' motives for sports differ across age and gender. It has been reported that those who are generally more than 65-years-old have a greater tendency to be attracted by extrinsic motives like awards, medals, and trophies. Results of studies that have examined masters athletes' motives for sport as a function of gender suggest that females are likely to place more value on intrinsic motivations such as personal enjoyment, health and fitness, and less value on extrinsic motives related to competition and goal achievement.

Another proposition from the research cited in this book is that a child-like outlook is the prerequisite for enjoyment of sports and serves as intrinsic motivation. This idea is partly in line with the results of several studies by Jean Côté and his colleagues. Côté suggests that early sports diversification, high amounts of play, child-centred coaches and parents, as well as being around peers who are in sports, are the main reasons why certain athletes invest a lot of effort and time into athletics later in life.

Finally, from a theoretical standpoint, major motivational theories including self-efficacy, self-determination, competence motivation, and the sport commitment model each imply that an individual's perception of his/her ability to perform a skill is the best predictor of enjoyment and intrinsic motivation.

How Can We Predict a Masters Athletes' Commitment to Sports?

The sport commitment model offers a unique approach to understanding why athletes continue their involvement in sport. Sport commitment is defined as a psychological state representing an individual's desire to continue participation in sports over time. The first type of commitment is *functional commitment*, which refers to the desire to continue with the target behavior because of volitional feelings of choice, or "wanting to" continue. The second type is called *obligatory commitment*, and is defined as the desire to continue with the target behavior because of feelings of obligation or because of "having to."

My colleagues and I have collected and begun to analyze data on sport commitment from masters athletes who participate and compete in a variety of sports including bowling, golf, marathon, and athletics. One of our repeated findings is that the athletes have high levels of functional commitment and moderate-to-low levels of obligatory commitment. This implies that masters athletes are committed to their sport primarily because they feel that they want to continue their participation, and to a lesser extent because they feel that they have to continue. This is important because research from other settings such as, youth sports, commitment in relationships, and commitment to work, as well as evidence from a number of interviews from this book, suggests that functional commitment is the healthier and more adaptive of the two types and is positively related to persistent training and participation behavior. With high levels of obligatory commitment, burnout and dropout are implicated.

In my investigation of each of the sports that we studied, I also found that enjoyment was the most consistent and the strongest predictor of functional commitment to sport. Of those in athletics and marathons, anticipation of future enjoyable experiences and decreased involvement in other attractive alternatives was also predictive of high functional sport commitment. Finally, for masters golfers, feelings of wanting to continue participating in their sport are enhanced by high social support from significant others such as the coaches, spouses, and/or training partners.

My research also discovered that, regardless of the masters sport, the most consistent and strongest predictor of high obligatory sport commitment was high expectations and pressure from significant others to continue participating. For masters athletes participating in golf and athletics, significant others play an even greater role. When athletes from these sports perceive that their participation is not supported by others who are important to them, their feelings of having to continue to participate heightens.

Altogether, diverse patterns of association between what de-termines commitment and the two types of commitment, sug-gest that the reliance on functional, as opposed to obligatory, type of commitment likely develops from diverse experiences with different sports. Still, one recurring finding was that sport enjoyment is an important determinant of both types of com-mitment. That sport enjoyment predicts functional commit-ment may not be surprising considering the voluntary nature of the sporting activities. However, in terms of the significance of sports enjoyment in predicting obligatory commitment, it could be that masters athletes feel that they have to continue their routine fitness programs in order to experience something that they enjoy doing, which is participating in their sport.

Can We Predict Masters Athletes' Passion for Sports?

Passion for sports may be defined as a strong inclination toward an activity that individuals love, is part of their identity, is con-sidered important, and is something in which they readily in-vest time and energy. There are two distinct types of passion that can be experienced for an athletic activity. One is obsessive passion, characterized by an internal motivational force that compels athletes toward an activity. Athletes who are runners that have this kind of obsessive passion report having no choice but to attend a scheduled running workout. With the other kind, called harmonious passion, people engage in their ath-letic activity willingly, knowing that they have a choice. Athletes with harmonious passion can easily put aside their workout if the need arises. Preliminary research has shown that obsessive passion is associated with negative emotional and behavioral consequences, while harmonious passion is related to positive consequences.

I recently surveyed 95 male and 43 female masters athletes and found that their scores were very high on harmonious pas-sion and moderate on obsessive passion. I also discovered that those who participated in sports for enjoyment reasons and because sports were part of their identity, were the ones who had a high sense of personal approval and the ability to choose to engage in their sport. For these masters athletes, sport involvement does not seem to overpower their identity or take over their personal lives.

Additional results suggest that masters athletes whose sport motives are internalized to help form their identities in a controlled manner, are the ones who have high levels of obsessive passion. They experience internal compulsions like guilt and/or anxiety if they cannot engage in their athletic activities. These compulsions lead them to participate in their sports at all costs – even when to do so can cause injury. As a result of the internal pressure they feel that causes them to engage so passionately in their activity, it is likely that these athletes who have high levels of obsessive passion find it extremely difficult to fully disengage from thoughts about their sport.

Consequently, these same athletes are much more likely to continue in their sport in spite of unfavorable circumstances, or when prevented from engaging in their sport, reflect on this and have negative feelings that border on psychological dependence. Dealing effectively with the latter may require strategies such as reassessing short- and long-term goals, cross-training and/or resting, spending more time working on mental skills, and thinking about, as well as, keeping up a training log.

Keeping Sports in Perspective

The value of keeping sports involvement in perspective is another key message communicated throughout this book. Maintaining this perspective can be achieved by placing an emphasis on health and well-being as major and desirable outcomes of participation, and by making sports a part of a well-rounded lifestyle.

Health and Well-being Are Preferred Outcomes of Participation

Despite the many positive experiences that we can get from masters sport participation, research shows that, for some, there are negative consequences to continued training and performing. These include experiencing feelings of desperation, trying to fix regrets and past failures, and bringing disruptions to the athletes' professional lives and to their families. For example, as mentioned before, studies show that masters athletes are more likely than younger athletes to experience acute and chronic injuries, have more fears of injury, and take longer to rehabilitate. Furthermore, in one of my studies, 80 percent of subjects reported having unfulfilled athletic goals that still exert considerable influence on their motivation to continue training and competing.

In another of the studies I conducted, most masters athletes reported that they would quit their sport only under extreme circumstances related to their health and well-being. 80 percent said that only an injury would make them stop; about 30 percent said that very old age and illness would prevent them from participating in sports, and 10 percent went so far as to say that they will never stop regardless of any condition. The following was a typical response, "I would not stop unless I was injured in such a way that I could not run upright." Again, understanding that the consequences of ignoring health and well-being could result in pain and even permanent injury may temper such extreme positions. Also, knowing how living such a narrowly focused life could lead to unhappy disconnection from others or from our work might influence our choices for a balanced life.

The knowledge we gain about how to continue to lead a long life of sports and activity can help us be aware of potential problem areas, and we can be better prepared to deal with challenges if they emerge. For some, this may require making the transition from a performance focus to a lifestyle focus. One useful strategy could include monitoring levels of involvement to make sure that sports do not take over a person's life and do not become his or her main priority. Masters athletes might also explore with their significant others, alternative perspectives on what their sport involvement could look like. To do this, they could switch to another sport for short periods of time, or if necessary, they could analyze advantages and disadvantages of modifying or leaving their sport. With longer life spans and a good quality of life at stake, it may be worth making adjustments to our points of view as we grow older.

In conclusion, results of the examination of 50 athletes over 50 provide an important stepping stone in research and in our understanding of optimal and healthy aging. The examples of those interviewed and the key messages about fitness found in this book are invaluable for those of us who want to maintain a healthy, athletic way of life as we age.

Chapter 10:
How Fast Do We Age?

by Dr. Vonda Wright, M.D.

Look around you the next time you race. If you are like most over-50 athletes, you will see a change happening; a paradigm shift. And it's not just that you are one of those who can remember life without cell phones. You also find that your age division is packed with lean, cut competitors, whose only indication that they are over-50 is a little grey hair and enough birthday candles to set a house on fire.

In the past five years, the world has been shocked by feats of endurance and shattered records set by older athletes, who have been categorized as out of the mold. Today, athletes from George Foreman to Lance Armstrong, from Dara Torres to Mark Marti, from Mark Recchi to Nolan Ryan, remind us that the older human body is capable of much more than we imagine. Tom Watson nearly claimed victory at the British Open, less than a year away from a total hip replacement, and just three years away from qualifying for social security.

But wait. Such amazing physical performance is not merely the privilege of elite masters athletes. It is the right of a growing number of older, high-performance athletes who can't be stopped. There is a tidal wave of motivated athletes who are determined to be strong and fit – even if they are over 50. They are proving themselves in all sports categories; showing us that older physiques are capable of more than we think they are.

Most orthopedic surgeons and many other medical profession-als have commonly held beliefs about the limits of our physical abilities as we age. It is thought that as our bodies grow old, they cannot heal as quickly, adjust to change as quickly, per-form as well in an event, or handle adversity as well.

While there are real physical changes that accompany aging, several key studies offer a rather different view; a view of older people with potential abilities that far exceeds our usual no-tions. If we had a better understanding of older adults' true po-tential abilities, we could be more supportive of their fitness goals. For example, valuing fitness options for older athletes dealing with medical issues would be a priority. We would hope that they would no longer just hear "quit that activity," with-out a discussion about how to preserve their fitness program, whether through modifications or by switching to another ac-tivity. And why is it that we too often hear that a medical patient is "too old" for a premium operation, so a temporary operation will suffice?

I have long believed that the perspective that aging is a slow decline from vitality to frailty is not the whole, or even the cor-rect, story. I believe that there must be factors that help masters athletes achieve success far past the time that we traditionally think of as peak performance. I want to understand what drives this success. Why is it that a 50-year-old male winner of the mile sprint is capable of finishing with an amazing 4:34 time? And how can a 70-year-old runner best a sedentary person half his age by doing a mile in seven minutes?

Much of the "slowing down" we see in the lives of older ath-letes can have more to do with choosing a sedentary life than anything else. For the last 43 years, I have watched my father Gene and his cronies fill their weekends with road races and had seen them thrive on competition. They marvel that they "still have it." Now 70, my father races most weekends and has several half marathons coming up this spring. When you look at pictures of him running cross-country in college and doing marathons now, the main difference is the amount of hair on his head. His well-trained legs and upper body look virtually the same. Why is this?

Why Research How Fast We Age?

Scientific studies of masters athletes are important because they can help lead our new, more active aging population to a stronger and more dynamic life. Studies can provide us with insights into how our bodies can age optimally. With a limited number of studies on the subject, lack of information also motivated me to conduct research on how age affects athletic performance. There is relatively little research that examines ways to slow or arrest what many think of as an inevitable decline from vitality to disability that accompanies aging.

We can start with the subject of our studies, and we do have a definitive subject: performance athletes. Through analysis of many different records, the older performance athlete is a model for successful aging. The typical master athlete trains for hours every day, over years and decades, and shows minimal-to-no age-related trends in body mass, composition, and physiology. Masters athletes and elite senior athletes give us the opportunity to review and compare physical performance at its crest, with smaller amount of variability than the general public. Studies often use highly trained athletes to determine human endurance and strength. Variables used include the human body's response to exercise and environmental stress, as well as heat, cold, and altitude. More important from a research standpoint, comparisons have been made between different groups of athletes, athletes of varying disciplines, and changes in performance over time.

Around 2003, I began studying masters athletes who participate in the National Senior Games (NSG). Masters athletics are for those over 40 years old, and NSG provides an opportunity for older athletes to participate in fitness and sports at local and national levels. I want to point out that all of the subjects in the studies we will review are normal people, not professional athletes. The recreational athletes involved in these games maintain high levels of physical functioning and a high quality of life throughout their life spans. Their mental outlook is bright, and most of them obviously embrace life joyfully and optimistically. They eagerly look forward to entering the next age category in their sport, because that gives them a chance to be even more competitive with a group that is mostly older than they will be.

Startling Running, Track and Field Performance Results

My first study, published in the *American Journal of Sports Medicine* in 2008, addressed these questions: who are these high-performing athletes, and when does aging really slow us down? I also wanted to know if there is a pattern to how we age, and when biology takes over no matter how active we are. To get answers, I looked at performance times of the top eight 2001 Senior Games finishers between the ages of 50 and 85, in track distances from 100 meters to 10 kilometers.

What I found startled me. Masters athletes' performance declined less than two percent per year for both men and women from age 50 to 75. Then, after the age of 75, something else happened. Their performance times suddenly dropped by eight percent per year. Why does performance plummet then? Is it due to cumulative factors like loss of muscle mass, flexibility, coordination, or is it diminished aerobic capacity that suddenly catches up with us?

To further evaluate trends, I studied American Track and Field record holders – the best of the best. I found that those from 30- to 50-years old had less than a one percent decline in performance, while the performance of those from 50- to 75-years old nearly doubled to just under two percent. Another sharp decrease in performance was seen in those over 75. These numbers were all consistent with my previous findings.

The following racing outcomes provide examples of these results. 24-year-old Sydney Maree set the men's collegiate record for a mile at 3:52.44 in 1981, but 35-year-old masters athlete Steve Scott, who clocked in at 3:54.13, was only two seconds behind Maree. We can also make an impressive comparison between 57-year-old Nolan Shaheed and an average 17-year-old that is in his prime. Whereas the teenager could have an 85th percentile running time of 6:06, Shaheed ran the mile much more quickly in 4:42.7. I also found several other studies that showed masters' groups running times were significantly improved compared with younger groups whose results plateaued. Clearly, well-trained, conditioned older athletes can be faster and more capable than most of us would have ever imagined.

Runners like these are great examples of the fact that *only 30 percent of how we age is determined by genetics, while the remaining 70 percent is determined by the lifestyle choices we make – including the choice to be active.* When using time, distance and speed to measure the performance of athletes, it is assumed that statistics are not skewed by potentially negative lifestyle factors like sedentary habits, smoking, and poor nutrition. At present, our genetic code cannot be altered, but training and lifestyle can.

Using training and conditioning programs as year-long activities rather than seasonal interludes is a big advantage for older athletes. Regular, dedicated exercise helps maintain endurance and strengthen our muscles. Training, as well as experience and a lifelong feel for the game, can also help masters athletes make significant achievements far past the time we traditionally think of them as having peak performance.

Age-related changes in endurance performance of marathon and half-marathon finishers were examined in another key study. They found that before age 50, there were no significant age-related losses in endurance performance; mean-marathon and half-marathon times were virtually identical in the 20- to 49-year-old age group. Moreover, age-related performance decreases of the 50- to 69-year-old subjects were only in the range of 2.6 to 4.4 percent range *per decade*. These, and other similar studies, show that the majority of older athletes who run are able to maintain a particularly high degree of endurance and fitness.

Weight Lifting, Swimming Performance Indicators Impressive

The study of records of older athletes is not limited to track and field or running events. Weightlifting records, analyzed over time, show approximately 1.0-1.5% per year in performance deterioration rates. While there is an incremental reduction in lifting ability over the years, this decline does not accelerate until after the age of 70.

One study found that in comparing muscle function in elite masters weightlifters with a healthy control group, muscle function declines at a similar rate with increasing age, but there are marked differences between the groups in the areas of strength and age. For tasks requiring muscular strength, an 85-year-old weightlifter was as powerful as a 65-year-old control subject.

After studying additional research results, the authors of the weightlifting studies came to several other conclusions that can help us understand what to expect of our strength and endurance as we age: (1) peak anaerobic muscular power, as determined by peak lifting performance, decreases progressively even from earlier ages than previously thought; (2) the overall magnitude of decline in peak muscular power appears to be greater in tasks requiring more complex and powerful movements; (3) the age-related rates of decline are greater in women than in men only in the events that require more complex and explosive power; and (4) upper- and lower-body muscular power demonstrate similar rates of decline with age.

In 1997 and 2003, Tanaka and Seals, leaders in the field of aging physiology, studied the performance of masters swimmers. Swimming studies have some advantages over running studies. Swimming is a non-impact activity with a lower rate of injury; so when trying to determine age-related performance decline, the age-related injury variable is automatically reduced in this sport. In addition, swimming has a more equal number of men and women who participate, making swimming studies representative of the male-to-female ratio in the general population.

To understand the relationship of age, gender, and swimming exercise task duration, Tanaka and Seals analyzed the peak exercise performance of swimmers, using results from the U.S. Masters Swimming Championships. Analysis of a 1,500-meter freestyle endurance event revealed peak performance levels in the 35- to 40-year-old age group until approximately 70 years of age. After 70, performances declined exponentially.

Compared with the distance event, performance in the 50-meter freestyle sprint showed a modest decline until age 75 in women and age 80 in men. The rate and magnitude of declines in both short- and long-duration swimming events with age were greater in women than in men. Findings indicate that the rate of swimming performance decline with advancing age depends somewhat on the length of the event that is selected and the gender of the person participating.

Swimmers fare significantly better than runners regarding the age at which rapid performance declines first appear. Whereas runners start to see rapid declines around 60-years-old, swimmers aren't affected until approximately age 70.

Biological Factors Affecting Performance in Older Athletes

Multiple age-related factors have been attributed to the performance decline seen in older athletes. These include declines in training intensity, reaction time, joint mobility, skeletal size, anaerobic and aerobic power supply, recovery ability, strength, endurance and coordination. Although we have no control over some of these factors, our motivation to train and our lifestyle choices give us control over some of them.

In addition, there are three key biological conditions that occur later in life that hamper athletic performance.

Loss of Aerobic Endurance Capacity

Age-related loss of aerobic endurance capacity is the factor that affects performance most, and loss of aerobic endurance capacity is one thing that cannot be improved with training. Reductions in maximal oxygen uptake or maximal aerobic capacity – called VO_2max – are a primary cause of decline in functional aging. VO_2max is a measure of how well the body absorbs and uses oxygen during exercise.

According to a number of studies, a reduction in maximal heart rate decreases VO_2max with age in either trained, or untrained, adults. The observed decline in VO_2max can be cut in half by intense regular exercise, but this effect is thought to be due primarily to improved cardiac output resulting from the body pumping more blood with each beat. Multiple studies have shown that there is no correlation between reduction in maximal heart rate and habitual exercise status.

Loss of Muscle Mass

A large reason for the loss of independence that we may have as we age is due to the loss of lean muscle mass. This condition is called sarcopenia. For most elderly people, the decrease in their muscle mass comes with an equal, or greater, decrease in strength and power. An increase in muscle weakness and fatigability also follows. We lose muscle power at twice the rate that we lose endurance capacity. We saw that endurance is lost at an average of 1.8 percent per year between the ages of 50 and 75, while muscle power is lost at 3.5 percent per year.

Muscle mass consists of the volume of muscle fibers present in a given muscle. Once a person's skeleton matures, no other fibers are created. As a result, change in muscle mass is a direct consequence of either a loss of the number of fibers, or a change in fiber thickness. It is unknown how much each factor contributes to muscle mass decline, and the role played by genetics and lifestyle is also unclear.

In any event, muscle loss can be modified by physical exercise. Even in people over 90-years-old, weightlifting can reverse some of the supposed age-dependent loss of muscle size, and loss of strength can be reversed as well. However, strength gains are modest compared to those of young individuals.

Loss of Exercise Economy

Changes in flexibility, joint motion, and coordination all contribute significantly to declines in exercise economy. When compared to their younger counterparts, shorter stride lengths and an increase in ground contact time are found in aged sprinters. The frequency of strides that an older person takes only shows a minor decline, however, and that may be due to lost muscle strength and power.

An often overlooked component to performance in older people is joint flexibility. With age, the body's connective tissue stiffens and knee motion decreases up to 33 percent. Joint flexibility helps maintain the ease with which we move, which in turn leads to more efficient motion. Stretching helps to improve joint flexibility as we grow older, and it also may reduce soreness after exercising.

For Older Athletes Lifestyle is Key to Performance

The studies that we read about were based on the observations of older performance athletes, who provide the best study models for examining how we age. Still, the lessons learned about the athletic abilities of these over-50 athletes, can be used by any who want to improve their own athletic performance as they age.

Having reviewed much of what is known about the effects of aging on older athletes, we know that 30 percent of performance is due to our genetic heritage and biological changes that are out of our control. Still, the remaining 70 percent is determined by the lifestyle choices we make, such as choosing to be active. In addition, many age-related issues affecting athletic performance later in life can be mitigated by smart training.

It's encouraging to know that in most sports, serious declines in functional performance are not observed until around the age of 70. Even after that, there is evidence that athletes can continue to expect good performance at an increasingly advanced age. It is also fascinating that those over-50 who participate in many high level sports continue to get faster.

The ranks of U.S. athletes who are over-50-years old are growing tremendously. They are not taking old age sitting down. They may be older, but they're not just watching from the sidelines. With steadfast dedication to their health, they are challenging themselves to be strong high-performers through wise fitness training. It really is a new era for athletes over 50 years old, and they still got game.

For more information, visit Dr. Wright's website at
www.vondawrightmd.com.

Chapter 11:
The Crew

"Ladies and gentlemen, my mother thanks you, my father thanks you, my sister thanks you, and I thank you!"

-George M. Cohan

Each one of the 50 over-age 50 athletes that I spoke with inspired this book. Whether they won many awards or no awards, their accomplishments are noteworthy because they have continued to integrate sports into their lives.

Every interview was important to the data and observations presented. Not having the space to include every interview in detail, I have tried to capture the essence of the remaining athletes in the following profiles. Their full interviews can be found at www.50athletesover50.com.

"Prepare for everything, fear nothing."
- Chris Scotto DiVetta

Chris Scotto DiVetta is a 52-year-old middle distance runner, who lives in Novi, Michigan. He has a demanding career as the chief operating officer of a major financial services company. Chris participated in track and field in high school and

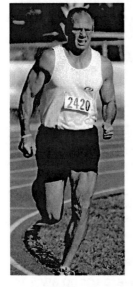

college, eventually achieving Division I All-American status. Early in his career, he stopped running altogether because he was tired of the sport and too busy at work. He was feeling discouraged because in order to improve, he needed to be able to spend more time in training.

When at his 30th high school reunion, an old schoolmate started riding him about how years ago he had run faster than Chris. The former schoolmate told him that he could even outrun him today. This piqued Chris' competitive spirit, so he challenged his friend to a race at the 50th annual Bishop Loughlin Games in New York. Chris convinced the organizers to add an alumni 400-meter race to the card, and with only a little preparation, he won the event in 55 seconds. The fire was lit and that was the beginning of Chris' masters running career.

Chris loves masters track and field, and is inspired by what the 70, 80, and 90-year old athletes can accomplish. He is currently preparing for this year's (2010) national championships, where he will retire from competitive running.

"Taking the lead is heaven, holding it is hell. Welcome to hell."

- Carl Bamforth

Fifty-one-year-old Carl Bamforth is a highly motivated, competitive inline distance speed skater, who lives in the "Garden City" of Victoria, British Columbia. Since age 16, Carl has participated in soccer, running, hockey, baseball, cycling, and triathlons, as well as inline skating. In his early forties, he developed plantar fasciitis from running, and was looking for other forms of exercise. A friend lent him a pair of inline skates, and he's been skating ever since.

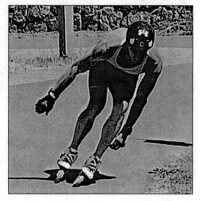

A single dad, Carl co-raised his daughter, who recently started college. He is a carpet and upholstery cleaning professional by trade, and prefers his active work to sitting at a desk. There are not many competitive skaters in Victoria, so most of the time he trains alone.

He is currently focused on setting the over-age-50 world records for the 1-hour, 6-hour, 12-hour, and 24-hour distance events. He has high hopes, because it will take a lot to beat John Silker's distance record for the 24-hour event, which is an unbelievable 282 miles. With great deliberation, Carl routinely does 50K-to-80K skates that take 2.5 to 4 hours, so that he can break the world records by such a margin that they won't be broken again during his lifetime.

"I'd rather design a prosthetic so someone can shoot a bow and arrow, or run as well as walk; not just enable someone to use a knife and fork."
- Bob Radocy

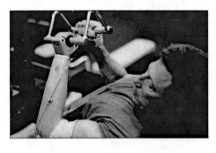

Bob Radocy is a 60-year-old archer and skier who lives in Boulder, Colorado. Bob had been active his entire life, playing baseball in high school and hunting with his father. Tragically, in 1971 he was involved in a car accident and lost his left arm just below the elbow. With a background in physical education as well as engineering, he was able to build himself a prosthetic arm that allowed him to re-engage in physical activities.

Following that success, he created TRS Inc., a company that specializes in developing such prosthetics. His prosthetic designs have helped thousands of people to participate in activities that make a huge difference for them. Some of the sports he's seen people take up are kayaking, lifting, climbing, running, and archery.

Whether he's practicing the sports he loves or witnessing a sunrise, Bob takes great pleasure in being outdoors. He told me he feels that one measure of the richness of a person's life is the number of sunrises he gets to see.

"I'm a journeyman."

- Bill Purves

Racewalking has shaped Bill's life in many ways. Through this sport, he has met his wife, enjoyed athletic success, lived in several countries, and learned their cultures. He has also has found racewalking to be the inspiration for his books.

Although he is quite accomplished in his sport, 65-year-old Bill Purves considers himself a lifelong journeyman; simply an experienced, reliable athlete. In high school, he ran cross-country, but was never one of the best runners. In college, he started racewalking when his coach told him that he didn't really need him in the running events, but he did need him to racewalk for additional team points. Nonetheless, Bill's record speaks for itself – he did win a place on the Canadian national racewalk team in 1971 and 1972.

This global citizen uses racewalking to build links between communities around the world. Bill now lives in Hong Kong, but has also lived in Newfoundland, Canada, and in Switzerland. In Hong Kong, he is well-known and goes by the handle Sahn Hahng Tai Bo, a Chinese name that he took when he moved there. Sahn Hahng Tai Bo is a character from a 14th century Chinese novel, who had the mystical ability to walk for hundreds of miles after invoking certain incantations.

Bill's most popular book is *China on the Lam*, which is about his 100-day walk through rural China. He is currently finishing a book called *Chinese Tortures* about his experience in adopting an extremely difficult training program used by the Chinese Olympic racewalkers.

"I'm intelligent. I know how to train. I perform the way I train. I believe in myself; and I'm feared by my competitors."

- Bret Williams

Fifty-year old Bret Williams is a long-time, talented, multi-sport athlete living in Grosse Point Park, Michigan. Over the years, he has participated in running, gymnastics, racquetball, handball, pole vaulting, and yoga. While he excelled at pole vaulting in high school and hoped to receive a college scholarship through it, a very bad ankle injury crushed that dream. Not a force to be stopped, Bret continued with athletics, eventually competing at a national level in racquetball and handball. In these competitions, he posed a significant challenge to professional players on more than one occasion.

When searching for employment, Bret came across a job posting for a pole vault coach at his former high school. Funny how it had once crossed his mind that someday he wanted to give back to the school and sport that meant so much to him. He snapped up the job and found himself with the desire to vault once again.

He now has his sights set on breaking the age 50-and-over world record of 15' 6 ¾" by the end of 2010. Not only does he see this as an opportunity to beat the best the world record, but also as a way to get over an injury that ruined his career plans 30 years ago.

When he was young, Bret found a couple other favorite sports through good ol' peer pressure. He started playing racquetball at age 14. One day, the friend that he played tennis with cut his tennis racquet off so that he could play the new game of racquetball. For a week or so, Bret refused to cut his own tennis racquet down, because he still liked to play the game. Finally, since he could not find anyone to play tennis with that week, he cut his racquet off too, and soon discovered that he loved the new game of racquetball after all.

The other sport that he found through his peers was handball. Often, when playing racquetball he was chided on the court by handball players who told him to put down the "sissy sticks" and play a real man's game. Being the versatile player that he is, he gave handball a try and found that he liked it, as well.

What gives Bret the edge? Flexibility, for one, as it keeps his athletic life fresh. Plus, a combination of tenacity, confidence in his own intelligence, and a thorough approach to training set him apart.

***

"Somewhere along the way I learned that having a goal is important. This advice applies to almost everything you do."

- Bruce Runnels

A sixty-year-old cyclist from Fort Collins, Colorado, Bruce Runnels has a background in law. He currently serves as an executive for The Nature Conservancy. Bruce played basketball in high school and ran cross-country in college. During those years, he also competed in canoe racing at state and national levels.

After college, Bruce ran road races and was considering doing a marathon when his life was changed by a serious car accident. His knee was badly hurt in the accident, making running very difficult. Not willing to give up exercise, Bruce discovered cycling and focused on that sport until work and family responsibilities took precedence.

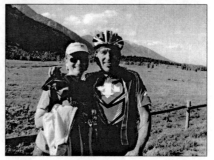

He left his bike in the garage for a few years, but eventually came to realize that he wanted to lose weight and needed to improve his level of fitness. Due to his knee injury, cycling was the only sport he could fully participate in. So Bruce dusted off the bike and went back to riding with a vengeance. He now trains for cycling competitions, and is very glad that he can still be fit and healthy through exercise.

***

"Good old-fashioned hard work."
- Don Sherrill

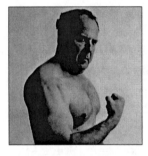

A retired environmental consultant, Don Sherrill is a 65-year-old power lifter who lives in Stone Mountain, Georgia. Don was sort of a skinny kid growing up, and didn't like the main sports of base-ball, basketball, and football. Although his school did not have competitive gymnastics, he did enjoy the tumbling shows his team put on during halftime at basketball games. Don also liked to water ski, and did some running in his thirties and forties when it was a "cool" thing to do.

When he was 64, he decided to start working out to get back in shape and help control some health issues that were creeping up on him. He joined a gym around the corner from his house, and in a short period of time found that he was bench-pressing some pretty heavy weights. Online, he discovered that what he was lifting was competitive for his age group. He decided to see what he could do in a "raw" competition in which the lifter lifts the bar purely under his own power.

He entered a meet and quickly bench-pressed 255 pounds, which was a national record as well as the meet record. His next goal is to bench-press 315 pounds, which he hopes to demonstrate or surpass in an upcoming meet. What happened to that skinny kid?

***

"It's true: no pain, no gain."
- Don Pratt

Don Pratt is a 76-year-old track and road runner who splits his time between Monticello, Illinois, and Fort Myers, Florida. While growing up in a coal mining town, Don played baseball, basketball, and track. After high school he played basketball until his son joined the cross-country team in the 7th grade. To help and inspire his son, Don started running with him and then became interested in running himself.

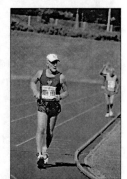

At this point, he has been running for 37 years and covers distances from 800 meters up to the half marathon. Don attributes his consistency and work ethic to growing up surrounded by hardworking people from the coal mines. Running is a family affair for him, since not only his son, but his daughter, son-in-law, and grandson also run. Don considers running with them to be top-notch family time.

***

"Be true to yourself."
- Ed Shaw

Ed Shaw is a 67-year-old cyclist and runner, who lives in Fort Collins, Colorado. Three years ago he retired from the civil engineering work that he relished. His last assignment was managing operations for a quarry in Newfoundland, Canada, which

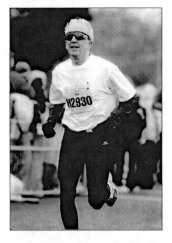

created jobs for 108 people who otherwise would have been out of work. Ed loved not only the good feeling that he got from helping these people, but also the satisfaction of doing his job well.

As evidenced by his victories in the challenging Mount Evans cycling race and the Austin Half Marathon, he brings that dedication for doing things well to his sports. Ed started cycling when urged by his son, who was a very good amateur cyclist. Ed found that he liked the feeling of speed when riding a bike, and that he had a talent for hill climbing. What's more, he has used his running and cycling skills in duathlons with good success. In recent years, he has been selective in choosing only the cycling races that he likes.

Gale Bernhardt, who I also interviewed for this book, told me about Ed and his ability to give it his all. She mentioned that on a recent ride with a group of very good cyclists, Ed demonstrated his cycling expertise by topping out first on a grueling hill climb in St. Vrain Canyon. He can't get enough of training, and treasures the friendships he has made through cycling and running.

***

"Nothing is written."

- Richard Stiller

A 64-year-old runner, Richard Stiller lives in the Santa Clara Valley of California. He works as a human resources consultant and has a degree in history.

He has reinvented himself several times during his running career. Having played soccer his first two years of college but not the last two, he ended up gaining a significant amount of weight.

When he completed college, Richard went on a strict diet and lost the excess weight, but found that he hated dieting. That's when he decided to reinvent himself and become a runner so that he could eat without guilt. At that time, the running boom was just getting underway. After running for a couple years, he ran his first race, called the Bay to Breakers. He finished the race at about 300th place, but this did not fit his image of himself.

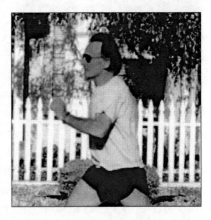

Two more reinventions followed. His next reinvention was going from a runner, to a serious, competitive runner. Being good at these kinds of transformations, Richard was soon ranked as one of the top runners in Northern California. He later found that the training regimen that had worked for him for many years, did not work for him in his forties, so reinvention number three was becoming a successful masters runner.

Richard is open to further reinvention and enjoys the process of recreating his athletic life. His remarkable outlook gives him many new opportunities and great success.

"If you're not having fun doing what you're doing, find something that's fun. And you shouldn't just do something for accomplishment, or to make someone happy."

- Gary Grobman

Gary Grobman is a 56-year-old-runner from Harrisburg, Pennsylvania, who played sandlot baseball in his youth, ran track in

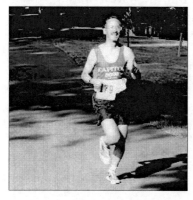 high school, and was back-up kicker on his college football team.

A college professor and author, Gary re-discovered track and field after he was hired to give management seminars to staff members of the national governing body for that sport.

He had to register for the conference in order to hold the seminars and be paid, and once a member, he started getting the mailings and newsletters. From these, Gary found out about the Mid-Atlantic Outdoor Masters Track Championship meet at Widener University in Chester, Pennsylvania. He got inspired to run the 5K, entered, and took 2nd place.

At that same meet, he also had his first and last encounter with the 3000-meter steeplechase, where he thought he might drown, so to speak. Gary has sworn off the steeplechase, unless lifeguards are on duty and he is allowed to wear a floatation device.

In the late 1970s and 1980s, Gary had a successful road racing career, and despite having a scary episode with his heart at the 2005 Boston Marathon, he continued to do track and field. In the summer of 2009, he dedicated himself to training for the National Senior Games in Palo Alto, California. There he won the bronze medal in the 5K and 10K road races, just seconds behind the first-place winners.

***

"Life should not be a journey to the grave with the intention of arriving in a pretty, well-preserved body; but rather to skid in broadside, in a cloud of dust, thoroughly used up, totally worn out, and declaring, wow, what a ride!"

- Jim Broun

Jim Woolvin Broun is a 57-year old-hurdler, who lives in Sarasota Florida, and once toured the country singing with the Woolvin James country music band that opened for artists such as Hank Williams Junior, Johnny Paycheck, and Alabama. Jim now works

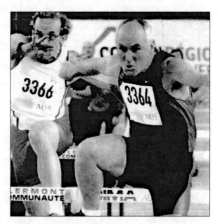

as a real estate investor. He played a number of sports for as long as he can remember. These included football, baseball, water skiing, snow skiing, cycling, and track.

When Jim was little he used to love to go watch the high school hurdlers when they practiced. Those hurdlers adopted Jim as a sort of mascot, and he first learned to hurdle when he was in elementary school. He hurdled throughout high school and college, until he got a recording contract and went on the road with his band.

In 2003 Jim, by chance, saw that a friend from college had won the masters world championship in the high jump, and this intrigued him. Online, he stumbled across masterstrack.com and saw the vibrant community of masters athletes. That's when he decided to hurdle once again. However, it wasn't going to be easy. It was a long road back, since he was carrying close to 200 pounds on his 5'9" frame. He worked hard to get back into shape, and in 2006 won the world indoor hurdle championships. Getting back into hurdling has changed Jim's life, and he can't live without masters track and field.

***

"I love my sports because of the gratification, fun, and satisfaction I get from them. I love the afterglow present after doing something that's really difficult."

- John Byrnes

Living in Fort Collins, Colorado, John Byrnes is a 54-year-old rock climber and skier. Growing up in Michigan, John swam, ran, and

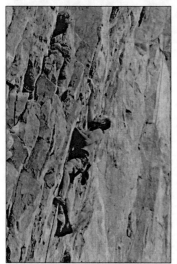

skied a bit, but his real athletic focus was bicycle racing. He proved himself early in his life by earning a three-time Michigan state champion title as well as a national ranking.

John gave up cycling during college because working to put himself through school was a priority. After college, his engineering career took him to Colorado where he was introduced to rock climbing by his then-girlfriend. He recalls that the very first climb he took, he was hooked. He also rediscovered skiing with his co-workers. John loves the feeling of accomplishment that he gets from doing these two sports. He marvels at how hard he works and how stressed he can feel during his exercise, yet when done, how self-satisfied he feels.

"What if?"

- Gary Leigh

Gary Leigh is a 54-year-old sprinter from Kennett Square, Pennsylvania, who had several very successful years in high school and college track and field. He was honored as Most Valued Player four years in a row, and looks back fondly on his 6th place finishes in the New York State high school track championships and in the junior college national championships. After college, Gary played and enjoyed volleyball and tennis for many years.

Following the breakup of his marriage 12 years ago, Gary went back to running track. Rekindling his joy of racing helped him through this tough period, and brought some happiness into his life.

In 2007, he placed second in the 100-meter event at the Senior Olympics in Louisville, Kentucky. He is now working his way back from a string of injuries that he suffered in 2008, and has his sights set on winning another medal at either the National Master Track and Field championships or the 2011 Senior Games.

What inspires Gary? He is competitive by nature and takes great joy in competing in masters track and field. He also loves the fact that every five years he gets rejuvenated when crossing into the next age group. He says that the camaraderie is also a draw, and that as he continues to get faster, he knows that he is still discovering his potential.

"Changing hearts, changing minds, changing lives."
- R.S. and Melody Mitchell

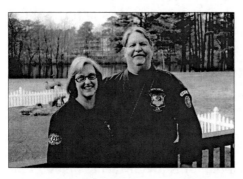 R.S. and Melody Mitchell, 61 and 54, live in Salisbury, Maryland, and own one of the largest martial arts schools in the country. R.S. learned martial arts from his father when he was very young. Melody got her start when at 34 she took a women's self-defense course from R.S. They are both devoted to bringing others these basic martial arts goals of self-esteem, self-control, self-discipline, self-defense, perseverance, respect for others, concentration, and physical fitness.

They have taught people from three years old and up. They offer classes for the very young that help them develop coordination and strength, as well as classes that teach older students how to defend themselves – sometimes with a cane. One of the best things about their studio is their success with students that have disabilities. They shared with me some of the astounding changes that they have seen in students with ADHD and physical handicaps.

One of their great pleasures is seeing others grow in confidence and discipline through martial arts. They appreciate that their sport keeps them physically and mentally fit, and feel fortunate that they have a sport they can practice together.

"Whether it's baseball, basketball, hockey, running or anything; just don't ever give up, stay focused on your goals, and keep pushing ahead."
- Scott Graham

Scott Graham is a 50-year-old endurance athlete who participates in running, triathlons, snowshoe racing, and anything else that can put his heart rate way up there. An executive for a financial services company, Scott lives in Westford, Massachusetts.

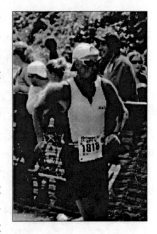

He discovered early on that he had enviable endurance when he finished first overall in a 25-mile walkathon. His walking training also benefited from his best buddy's father, a marathoner who would bring the boys to run with him when he did warm ups.

Scott has run 23 consecutive Boston Marathons, and most recently ran 3:01, just missing the three-hour mark. He is known in his local running club as PHAT, for Pain Heavy At Times, a reference to his propensity to push though pain levels that would stop most others.

Despite the challenge of fitting his training into his busy life, he is dedicated to athletics. Due to his demanding job, he often works out at 4 a.m. He enjoys using his gift of stamina, thrives on working out, and is happy to have his network of athlete friends.

"Skating was such a blast when I was a kid, running around on skates with my sisters and my dad...then to come back to it later in life was like discovering it all over again, but in new ways."

- Suzy Devers

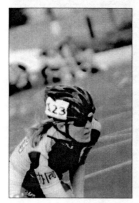

A 57-year old ice and inline speed skater, Suzy Devers lives and writes in Louisville, Colorado, but she grew up on the East Coast where she ice skated from age five with her sisters and father. Throughout the years, Suzy played other sports, and in her thirties began inline skating for fun and exercise.

Her love for ice skating re-emerged at age 52, and she started looking for a pair of speed skates for the ice. It was hard to find ice skating equipment in Colorado, but her quest put her in touch with an inline skating coach in Boulder, Colorado. She wound up buying inline skates and went on to skate a variety of distances on the road, indoors, and on a banked track. She eventually found ice skates and continued to skate on ice, too.

One of the things that draws Suzy to her sport is the variety of forms that skating can take. She also loves how it reminds her of the fond memories that she has of skating when she was a child.

"Difficulty and suffering are prerequisites for fulfillment."

- Don Ardell

Don Ardell is a 71-year-old-triathlete who lives in St. Petersburg, Florida. In 2009, he won the US National Sprint Triathlon Championship in Newport Beach, Virginia, and the World Sprint Triathlon Championship on the Gold Coast of Australia for his

age group. Growing up in Southwest Philadelphia, Don played all kinds of games. In high school, he ran track and cross-country.

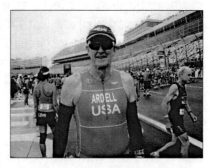

He joined the U.S. Air Force straight out of high school, and managed to earn a spot on base with the All-Air Force teams for football, basketball, baseball, volleyball, softball as well as running track as a miler. Don did anything he could to stay off KP (kitchen patrol), and performed the boring duties of a lowly airman so that he could attend night classes for college credits. That is, when he was not off representing one air base team or another in sports.

Don was observed by a college basketball scout during an Air Force tournament, and that led to his eventual acceptance at George Washington University on a full basketball scholarship. With credits accumulated from his night classes during his Air Force years, he started college as a sophomore. This made it possible for him to take a lighter academic load so that he could play varsity basketball, act in student theater and musical comedy productions, and chase coeds – one of whom he married.

After completing graduate school at the University of North Carolina at Chapel Hill with a degree in urban planning, Don took up competitive handball. Playing throughout his thirties, he won many titles, including the Minnesota state championship. Entering his forties, Don discovered road running. Five years later, and after many marathons, he moved from the San Francisco Bay Area to Orlando to teach at a university and manage a wellness center.

His introduction to triathlons happened as a consequence of his work. He was the featured speaker at a hospital wellness conference in Kansas City, and while there, he was asked to promote his wellness lectures by conducting an athletic event. On a borrowed bike and with the help of all kinds of swimming aides just shy of water wings, Don survived the encounter. He managed to finish the ordeal almost, but not quite last – thanks to his strong running ability. That experience fascinated Don, and in time, he learned how to swim properly and ride a bike competitively.

Don is credited with writing the first popular book to jumpstart the wellness movement. It is called *High Level Wellness: An Alternative to Doctors, Drugs and Disease*, published by Rodale Press in 1976. Since then, he has written 15 other books and delivered hundreds of presentations at hospitals, worksites and conferences throughout the U.S. as well as 16 other countries. His newsletter, the *Ardell Wellness Report*, has been circulated globally since 1984, and more than 500 editions have been produced and distributed.

***

"Live today the way you would like to in the future."
- Weia Reinboud

A native of the Netherlands, Weia Reinboud is a 59-year-old high jumper and javelin thrower. A student of physics, sociology, philosophy, graphic design, and nature photography, she has a keen interest in learning. In her youth, Weia was an 800-meter runner. She took a twenty-nine-year hiatus from athletics before choosing the high jump as her new sport. At age 45, she was in a sort of mid-life crisis, and was watching the European track and field championships when she noticed how lean, long, and slender all of the athletes were.

Wanting to look and feel better, Weia thought that maybe she would just try sports again. Unaware of the masters athletics movement, she didn't expect much of herself. She was completely surprised that in her first year, her performance matched the Dutch national record in the high jump. Within five years, she had set the world high jump record.

Weia has also achieved success in the heptathlon as well as the double heptathlon, in which she still owns the world record. At age 55 she took up javelin throwing, and now hopes to break the world records in both the high jump and the javelin when she crosses into the 60+ age group next year.

***

"Whether you think you can or whether you think you can't, you're right."

- Stephen Black

Stephen Black is a 57-year-old triathlete who lives in Lafayette, Colorado, where he combines his passion for athletics with his physical therapy profession. In high school, Stephen dabbled in baseball, basketball, and football, but when he saw a gymnastics exhibition, he knew he had found something he'd love. In high school and college, he enjoyed success with the sport. Shortly after he graduated from college, he took up running

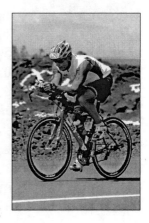

and was introduced to triathlons by a friend.

He says that one of his greatest achievements was his successful transition from being a college athlete to someone with a healthy, active lifestyle. Having his father die from a massive heart attack at age 62, and seeing how his mother bravely lived with rheumatoid arthritis, Stephen developed the motivation and the will to make the Performance-to-Lifestyle transition.

***

"In order to run fast, you have to run fast."
- Jim Morton

Jim Morton is a 54-year-old 400- and 800-meter runner who lives in Springfield, Massachusetts. Jim has participated in

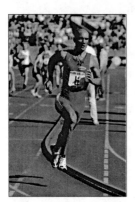

sports since he was five or six years old. Track, triathlons, and boxing were his primary interests. In high school, Jim always wanted to be a 400-meter runner, but there were many runners faster than him.

When he was 49, he figured maybe those guys were gone and that he could be a competitive 400-meter masters runner now. He actually found there were still quite a few masters 400-meter runners ahead of him, but that he really was one of the fastest 800-meter runners in the country.

Jim is a lawyer by profession, but he became the president and chief executive officer of the Greater Springfield YMCA, which works to improve the lives of its youth. Jim and his coworkers established an indoor track team for inner-city kids that enable them to train and compete through the winter months. This allows them to be more competitive in the spring season. Terrific personal success stories resulted from the track team, including Massachusetts state champions, New England champions, and qualifiers for the Junior Olympics.

In 2005, Jim donated two thirds of his liver to a lifelong friend. Afterwards, he worked long and hard to get back in shape. Currently, he is focused on winning the 2010 World Indoor and Outdoor 800-meter championships. He also hopes to run the 400-meter as part of a relay team at the World Championships.

Page 166: John Byrnes photo by Kirk Donaldson.
Page 174: Jim Morton photo by Cheryl Treworgy of PrettySporty.com.

Epilogue:
The Road Forward

"If you come to a fork in the road, take it."
-Yogi Berra

Recently, I was out for a run and thinking about a comment someone made to me the previous day about being "Over the hill." I was considering what that meant, when I got a visual of one long, steady hill that crests and then descends. The more I thought about this as an analogy for life, the more ridiculous it seemed. For me and all the athletes that I interviewed, life is an up-and-down, three-dimensional landscape peppered with an incredibly complex and diverse terrain. The analogy of one, long steady climb and decent, didn't seem to fit.

I think back about the hills that I've climbed. Some were thrust upon me and some I chose. When I was seven years old, my father died of lung cancer, which was a hill I definitely had not chosen. I have also chosen my share of hills. I chose to go to school, get married, write a book, climb Washington's Column in Yosemite, be a competitive runner, change jobs, get divorced, learn to play the banjo, get remarried...you get the idea. One way or another, we all have hills to climb.

Superimposed on this complex landscape of life, is the path of chronological aging that we all march further along. I do not plan on going down this road quietly. I will go running, jumping, climbing, laughing, and singing – all with as much energy as I can muster. What makes it all the more joyous for me, is that through interviewing 50 athletes over 50 and through writing this book, I have an even better backpack full of tools, insights, and stories of friends to help me along the way.

I set out to hear from a cross-section of older athletes how I could continue to enjoy good health and a high quality of life throughout my life. In studying their histories, I have learned what can help and what can hinder my fitness journey. I now have a better understanding of what motivates older athletes, and when moving my body – I will tap into my pure instinct to play.

Like a kid, I will encourage myself to have fun with exercise and sports, and I will be alert to other responsibilities that can crowd fitness out of my schedule. Since a consistent exercise routine is so important, I will also be alert to potential injury that can disrupt my routine. To avoid injury, I will treat my body well and be somewhat cautious about working my fitness program.

By using these tools, I know that I stand an even better chance of staying strong and healthy as I grow older. Resting in the knowledge that the 50 athletes supplied, I understand that as I establish fitness as a lifestyle, my success is naturally fueled by the joy that I get from playful movement, good health, accomplishment, and athletic companionship.

With lessons garnered from the stories we heard, I hope that you will join me down the raucous road of life. I hope that you don your backpack, grab your songbook, and meet me at a trailhead. Our paths will lead us on very different adventures, but I hope we can meet up occasionally to share stories and marvel at our strength and good health.

Happy trails!

ABOUT 50 INTERVIEWS

Imagine a university where not only does each student get a text book custom tailored to a curriculum they personally designed, but where each student literally becomes the author!

The mission of *50 Interviews* is to provide aspiring, passionate, driven people a framework to achieve their dreams of becoming that which they aspire to be. Learning what it takes to be the best in your field; directly from those who have already succeded. The ideal author is someone who desires to be a recognized expert in their field. You will be part of a community of authors who share your passion and who have learned firsthand how the *50 Interviews* concept works. A form of extreme education, the process will transform you into that which you aspire to become.

50 Interviews is an ever expanding collection of books, CDs, videos, and software that serve to inform, educate, and inspire others on a wide range of topics. Timely insight, inspiration, collective wisdom, and best practices derived directly from those who have already succeeded. Authors surround themselves with those they admire, gain clarity of purpose, adopt critical beliefs, and build a network of peers to ensure success in that endeavor. Readers gain knowledge and perspective from those who have already achieved a result they desire.

If you are intersted in learning how you can become an author (no writing skills necessary!), I would be more than happy to provide you all the details and brainstorm potential topics with you. You can contact me via email at: 50interviews@gmail.com, by phone: 970-215-1078 (Colorado), or through our website:

www.50interviews.com

All my best,
Brian Schwartz
Authorpreneur and creator of *50 Interviews*

OTHER 50 INTERVIEWS TITLES

Additional topics based on the 50 Interviews model that have already been released or are in development:

Professional Speakers
By Laura Lee Carter and Brian Schwartz

Successful Jobseekers
By Gordon Nuttall

Young Entrepreneurs
By Nick Tart

Artists
By Maryann Swartz

Video Marketing Pioneers
By Randy Berry

Attraction Marketers
By Rob Christensen

Spiritualists
By Tuula Fai

Parents
By Victoria Edge

Scientists
By David Giltner

Wealth Managers
By Allen Duck

Millionaire Women
by Kirsten McCay-Smith

Entrepreneurs
by Brian Schwartz

Property Managers
by Michael Levy

Physicians
by Rich Fernandez

Learn more at
www.50interviews.com

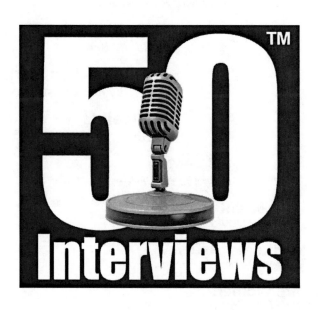

CPSIA information can be obtained
at www.ICGtesting.com
Printed in the USA
LVOW10s1051111217

559351LV00014B/126/P